THE
DUKAN DIET

Made Easy

Cruise Through Permanent Weight Loss— and Keep It Off for Life!

Dr. Pierre Dukan

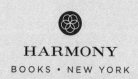

HARMONY

BOOKS · NEW YORK

Contents

Introduction

For over forty years, every day in my work as a doctor I have been fighting weight problems. Starting out on my own, I first crafted my skills by working with individual patients in consultations. While still a very young doctor, I was fortunate to devise the protein diet. As the years went by I improved it, adjusting it based on my patients' feedback and needs. Gradually the diet turned into a comprehensive program, which was published in France in 2001 as *Je Ne Sais Pas Maigrir (I Can't Lose Weight)*. Since then, and giving me the greatest rewards imaginable, more than 8 million readers in over twenty countries have read this book. Unfortunately, I do not know how many have followed the diet suggested and, even less, how many have attained their True Weight, consolidated it, and, most important, never put any weight back on.

However, I do know that every day I receive an ever-growing number of heartfelt messages from readers who, because they have lost weight using this book and its method, go out of their way to let other people know about it. My method spread simply by word of mouth, without any advertising to back it up. Nowadays, I am conscious that I am no longer the sole owner of my method; it also belongs to my readers who follow it and recommend it to others.

Who are they? Mostly they are well-organized women, writing from all over the Internet world. To date, over 500 sites, forums, and blogs have been listed where anonymous contributors and volunteers share their experiences of controlling their weight with my diet. It was these women who eventually named my method after me. I would never have dared do that myself.

This book and method are aimed at people who want to lose weight but, faced with the overwhelming choice of diets now available, do not know which one to choose. According to my records, there have been 210 diets developed since the 1950s, of which 72 have been published. Only 15 have any coherence, and they can be boiled down to 6 main programs:

- **The low-calorie diet** is the oldest and, in theory, the most logical, but in practice the least effective diet.
- **Atkins** was revolutionary and effective, but it leaves the door wide open to fats and cholesterol.
- **Weight Watchers** meetings were very innovative, but its low-calorie diet does it a disservice.
- **The South Beach Diet** is a good diet, but it lacks any proper stabilization.
- **The protein powder diet** is sold throughout the world, but it is the most unnatural diet. Once dieting is over, it leads to a massive and permanent weight explosion.
- **The method that I suggest, aka the Dukan Diet**

I have trouble writing this as it may appear immodest, but I really do believe that, to date, of all the diets put forward, my method is by far the best. It is set out simply; it provides a solid framework; it is effective; you start getting immediate results and these results last. Its 100 as-much-as-you-want foods are all natural foods, and its concept is simple; it is easy to follow, and it can tackle all weight-loss situations. For all these reasons, it seems to me to be the best way we have at the moment of losing weight and, most important, of not putting weight back on again.

Sylvia W.—Lost 24 pounds

Go for it; it really is a wonderful, easy, enjoyable diet. You won't regret starting it.

I am campaigning for this method to become a standard benchmark in the worldwide fight against weight problems. Readers, I am asking you to judge how well it works. In this book, you will find my entire method, along with an introduction to physical exercise, which I now prescribe as I would medication, and a recipe section so that while you diet you can make all sorts of different dishes (this edition includes new vegetarian recipes).

Recipes provide pleasure, and without pleasure our struggle against weight problems would be about restriction and nothing else.

So go off to do battle with these three pointers to encourage you: as much as you want of the allowed foods, fast results, pleasure in your food!

Are you up for it? Let yourself be guided—your scale is shaking already!

A TRIED-AND-TESTED METHOD

What is the only food group that is low in calories and leaves the body full and satisfied without making it feel tired? Proteins.

The story behind this diet

It all started when I was a young general practitioner working in Montparnasse in Paris. One of my patients was obese, and he seemed to have come to terms with it. However, one day he booked an appointment and asked me to help him lose weight. At first I replied that I was not a specialist in the field. He countered straightaway that he knew all the specialists I was referring to very well and that he had tested all the existing methods without ever managing to lose any weight for any length of time.

Sounding deeply disheartened he told me, "Since my teens I have gained and lost hundreds of pounds!" Then he added, "I'll follow your instructions to the letter. I'll do whatever you want except for one thing—don't stop me from eating meat. I just love meat too much!"

When I immediately shot back the reply, "All right, eat only meat, as much meat as you want for five days," that was how the adventure started.

The following week, my patient was back in my office, but this time he was beaming. He had lost almost 11 pounds!

So we both agreed to continue with the experiment. However, I did ask him to ensure he was drinking enough water and to have a blood test, because I was worried about his cholesterol. One week later, his blood test results were absolutely fine, and he had lost another 4 pounds . . .

I then started studying in greater detail how proteins could usefully contribute to a weight-loss diet. After twenty days of dieting, my patient had lost over 21 pounds, but he was now beginning to grow weary of his favorite food. So we added a few vegetables to his meals, along with some dairy products, eggs, and fish. As for quantities, I continued to avoid any restriction. He greatly enjoyed this freedom, and at the same time, he graciously stuck to my very precise instructions about eating only proteins and a few vegetables.

Since then, as you will see from reading these pages, the method has been fine-tuned thanks to feedback from my patients, and I have created some simple, easy recipes. However, the basis of the diet has not changed—by eating proteins it is possible to lose weight quickly, permanently, and without restricting quantity.

With the advent of the Internet, I really can combine my experience with that of my patients. The people who visit my site share their experiences with me; my tips merge with their tips; and the women writing on the forums add their own recipes, less professional but just as creative, to my recipes. We work together toward a common goal, which is to lose weight while enjoying eating! This book is therefore the end product of many long years of experiments, tests, and developments that you can benefit from today.

If, like my first patient, you follow to the letter the instructions that follow, it will be impossible for you not to lose weight quickly. You do not need any complex equipment, just a bathroom scale. You don't need to count calories, weigh food, or use any tables with complicated figures.

Reading about the different stages of the diet is very easy because you only have two or three instructions to memorize. As for everything else, within this simple structure, you can eat as much as you want.

However, before we start examining the principles behind the diet itself, we need to quickly remind ourselves about the different food groups so that you avoid making mistakes when selecting your ingredients.

Carbohydrates, fats, and proteins

All the different foods we eat are made up of just three categories of nutrients: carbohydrates, fats, and proteins. The caloric value of these three groups is different. However, we know today that it is important not to judge a food solely by the number of calories it provides, since the body does not deal with the 100 calories contained in a piece of chocolate cake, fish, or a salad dressing in the same way. How many of these calories the body ends up extracting varies greatly, depending on where they come from. This is why sound knowledge of these nutrients is important to have so that you can make the right choices with the diet.

Andy C.—Lost 40 pounds (did the diet with his wife)

Stick with it faithfully, and you will be rewarded for your efforts.

Carbohydrates

Carbohydrates can be divided into "fast sugars" and "slow sugars." Fast sugars are the sugars found in sweet-tasting foods such as candy, cakes, wine, honey, fruit, and so on. Everyone knows that a dieter must avoid them, especially since soon after assimilating fast sugars we feel really hungry again. Bread and pasta as well as legumes such as lentils and dried beans contain slow sugars. These are called slow sugars because the body takes longer to assimilate them than fast sugars. As far as our metabolism goes, fast sugars encourage insulin secretion, which in turn makes the body produce and store fats.

Carbohydrates only provide 4 calories per gram, but we tend to eat them in considerable quantities to feel full.

Our diet's program cuts out carbohydrates until you get down to your target weight (except for the carbs found in vegetables, oat bran, and fat-free dairy products). During the Consolidation period (Phase 3) carbohydrates—bread and starchy foods—are reintroduced. Then during Stabilization (Phase 4), you will be completely free to eat them again six days out of seven.

Fats

Dieters usually recognize fats as their number one enemy if they are hankering after a slim figure. They are virtually absent from our program apart from what is found in the meat and fish you are allowed to eat. Fats can come from animals; cooked meats contain a lot of fat as do mutton and lamb. Some poultry and fish also have a very high fat content, for example, duck, goose, salmon, tuna, etc.; however, because they contain a lot of omega-3, fats from "oily fish" are good for our health and protect the heart. Full-fat butter and cream are, of course, not allowed.

Although vegetable fats such as olive or walnut oil are beneficial for your health (they are particularly rich in omega-3 fatty acids and good for your heart), they will also be banned throughout your diet, except for up to a teaspoon for a vinaigrette mixture or ⅛ teaspoon of oil to grease a pan.

Carolyn M.—Lost 18 pounds

Don't worry that you will be constantly
hungry, you won't. Just do it!

Proteins

Of the three food groups, proteins are the only one that is not a natural energy source for the body. The body uses proteins for building (growth), for example by growing new skin, nails, hair, and muscle tissue. The body also uses proteins to maintain and repair itself, for example by maintaining memory and producing blood cells, etc.

Proteins also play a role in how the immune system functions. Proteins are composed of a collection of twenty different amino acids and are found in animal products and vegetables.

Animals provide us with the best source of proteins. Some foods contain a lot of protein but virtually no fats and so are especially useful for our diet; such foods, for example, include lean cuts of beef, turkey, certain organ meats, white fish, shrimp, crab, and tofu. Egg white is the benchmark protein and contains no cholesterol, which is concentrated in the egg yolk. You can create a never-ending range of tasty, filling recipes using egg whites.

Cereals and legumes also contain proteins, but these proteins have too many carbohydrates, which is why they are not included in our diet. During the Attack phase, your menus must be made up of proteins, and only proteins.

Proteins—a vital nutrient

It is not dangerous to eat only proteins as part of a diet—quite the opposite in fact, since proteins form the only group of nutrients that your body cannot synthesize on its own. By drawing upon its reserves, your body will find the carbohydrates and fats it needs for energy. However, it is incapable of making proteins itself, which is why a diet lacking in proteins may be dangerous. Whenever there is a shortage, the body takes the proteins it needs for its survival from its muscles, skin, and even its bones. A diet must therefore always provide at least 1 gram of protein per day for every pound of lean body mass and proteins should be evenly distributed over the day's three meals.

What proteins do (backed up by scientific evidence)

Pure proteins reduce your appetite

Since proteins are not easily digested, they are powerful appetite suppressants. Indeed, eating a good amount of pure proteins makes your body secrete "ketones," which will give you a lasting feeling of satiety. After three days of eating pure proteins, hunger disappears completely. As you are no longer racked by hunger, you can resist snacking more easily.

By digesting proteins you burn more calories!

Digesting proteins is an extremely lengthy process. Did you know that it takes over three hours to digest and assimilate a high-protein meal? But this is not all. In order to extract calories from proteins, the body has to work very hard indeed. It has been calculated that to get 100 calories, 30 of them are used up! Just having to digest a high-protein meal reduces the calories it provides.

Remember to drink lots of water to get rid of waste

The body uses only some of the proteins it is given. Just 50 percent can be assimilated; the rest is eliminated as waste in your urine and may lead to an increase in uric acid. To offset this minor inconvenience, all you need to do is make sure that you drink enough throughout the diet (1½ to 2 liters of water per day). Our studies show that if sufficient water is drunk, eating proteins poses no particular risk. This proteins + water combination is even very beneficial in flushing out cellulite!

Eating pure proteins cuts down your calorie intake

For human beings, the ideal proportion for nutrients (enabling us to extract as many calories as possible for our survival) is the following formula: 5 parts carbohydrates and 3 parts fats to 2 parts proteins. When our food intake matches this ratio, this is ideal for assimilating nutrients, and they are assimilated through the small intestine with maximum efficiency. Once these proportions are reversed, the way the body absorbs its calories is also disrupted, which can be put to particularly good use as part of a diet. Limiting what we eat to just one of the three food groups automatically results in calories being less well absorbed. However, eating only carbohydrates or fats is inconceivable as it would endanger your health in the long term by increasing cholesterol and causing diabetes and cardiovascular complaints. A diet based on a single food group without putting your body at risk is only possible with proteins. Give your digestive system protein meals and it will struggle to extract all the calories contained in the food. So the body will then attempt to take only the proteins it absolutely needs to maintain its organs, making very little use of the remaining calories available.

Pure proteins help you combat water retention

Diets based on plants, fruits, vegetables, and mineral salts encourage water retention. The Dukan Diet, which is based on proteins, is quite the opposite. It is water-repellent, promoting the elimination of urine, which is especially useful during menopause or if you are simply premenstrual. Our program is therefore very beneficial for women who tend to retain water more easily in their tissues. Some of my female patients, with little experience of being overweight before menopause, unexpectedly find themselves with swollen ankles, heavy legs, and a bloated stomach. All of a sudden, the odd bit of dieting they had tended to rely on throughout their lives (for example, eating carefully after a week of festivities) no longer has any effect. Our diet's Attack phase, with proteins and nothing else, works miracles for them.

Stephanie T.—Lost 18 pounds

Go on the diet with someone who will help you stay strong on your weak days.

Proteins are an effective way of tackling cellulite

The results of a Dukan high-protein diet on cellulite are spectacular. Quite simply, these results can be explained by the water-repellent effect of proteins and the intense filtering of the kidneys. Water goes into tissues and comes out again full of waste matter. The cellulite is cleaned out. This is why, and we will keep on saying it, drinking lots of water throughout the diet is crucial.

Andy I.—Lost 70 pounds

It's worth it!!!

The Dukan Diet

How is the Dukan Diet organized?

At the outset, the diet was called "Protal," a contraction of two words: proteins and alternatives. It was a diet duo that worked like a two-stroke engine with a pure protein diet period, the Attack phase, followed by a period of proteins combined with vegetables, because the body needs time to recuperate so that it can digest its weight loss. My readers have since then done me the honor of associating my name with this diet: the Dukan Diet.

Afterward, thanks to the experience that I shared with my patients, I realized that this program was not quite enough. Once they had lost weight and achieved their goal, my patients actually showed an extremely great propensity for just letting it all go and for quickly putting back on the weight they had just lost. Which is why today, the Dukan Diet is part of a complete weight-loss program, made up of four phases that are not to be separated from one another. If you follow them one after the other and as a complete package, you are guaranteed not to put weight back on. Likewise you are also guaranteed to regain weight if you do not follow the final two phases: Consolidation and Stabilization.

The Dukan Diet offers certain advantages, and your motivation is bound to remain high, for four reasons:

- The Dukan Diet gives you a list of very precise instructions; to succeed all you have to do is follow them.

- The Dukan Diet is a completely natural diet. Of all the natural diets, it is the diet that produces the best results.
- The Dukan Diet does not cause frustration, since you can eat as much as you want of its 100 foods.
- You cannot follow the Dukan Diet halfheartedly—either you succeed and agree to everything, or you fail!

Shawn E.—Lost 25 pounds

It is something you have to want—nobody else's goals will do.

The four main phases in the Dukan program

Phase 1: Attack phase with pure proteins
This phase only uses high-protein foods. It is very short; weight loss is very quick and highly motivating.

Phase 2: Cruise phase: proteins + vegetables
This is how you will achieve your target weight: your True Weight. This initial period in which you have started to wage war on your surplus pounds is followed by a "Cruise" period, during which you opt for a diet of alternating days of pure proteins with days of vegetables + proteins. This will allow you to reach your chosen weight.

Phase 3: Consolidation phase
Once you have gotten down to the weight you wanted, it is important to avoid the "rebound phenomenon"—after rapid weight loss, the body tends to pile back on any lost pounds extremely quickly. This is therefore an especially tricky period, and under no circumstances is the diet over yet. For every pound you have lost, you will need to remain 5 days in the Consolidation phase.

Phase 4: Stabilization phase

You have to adhere to three simple, essential measures for the rest of your life, in particular to Protein Thursdays, a sentinel day that stands guard over the six other days of the week. The Permanent Stabilization phase is every bit as crucial because it is decisive in determining the success of your diet. So that you do not put back on any of the weight you have lost, you will have to apply some simple measures throughout your life. One day a week you must follow the Dukan Diet's Attack phase to the letter, preferably every Thursday. Having to do this will protect you from regaining weight.

As you can see, the Dukan Diet takes care of you so that you are never ever left to cope on your own again.

SLIMMING SECRET #1—
APPLE CIDER VINEGAR

Several studies suggest apple cider vinegar helps with weight loss. The recommended amount is 2 tablespoons. Taken at the start of a meal, vinegar helps break down proteins and fats. The acidity can sometimes limit how much a person can consume— those with a sensitive stomach or past history of ulcers should not use it at all.

Vicky T.—Lost 75 pounds

You're never too old to lose the weight.

The diet's four phases

PHASE 1

The Attack phase with pure proteins (PP)

This is the most motivating period because you will see your weight drop with breathtaking speed, a little as if you were fasting. This Attack phase is a real machine of war.

During this phase you are going to eat the purest possible proteins, while cutting out all other foods as much as possible. In reality, it is not possible to eliminate carbohydrates and fats altogether from what you eat. In fact, apart from egg whites, no food is made up entirely of protein. Therefore your diet will bring together a certain number of foods whose composition is as close as possible to pure protein, including, for example, some categories of meat, fish, shellfish, poultry, eggs, and fat-free dairy products.

Length: This period can last between 1 and 7 days, depending on how much weight you have to lose.

PHASE 2

The Cruise phase: pure proteins (PP) alternate with proteins + vegetables (PV)

This second phase works together with the first one, and thus they cannot be separated from each other. You are going to alternate periods of proteins + vegetables with periods of pure proteins.

Just like the first phase, this second one allows you the same complete freedom regarding quantities. Both phases let you eat "as much as you want" of the foods allowed, at any time.

Later on we will look at how you alternate these two phases, which will depend on how much weight you have to lose, your age, and also your motivation.

Length: You must follow this Cruise phase without any breaks until you reach your desired weight.

PHASE 3

Consolidating the weight you have slimmed down to

The purpose of this phase is to get you eating more foods again and to stabilize your weight. You will be able to eat a greater variety of foods, but you need to avoid the rebound effect and the risk of regaining weight. Your body will try to resist, even more so if you have just lost a considerable amount of weight. Given that its reserves have been plundered, your body will now react by attempting to build up some new reserves. To do this, it will cut down as far as possible the amount of energy it uses, and it will absorb as much as it can from any food you eat. During this period, a copious meal that would have had little impact at the start of the diet will now have far-reaching repercussions.

This is why the quantities of richer foods will be limited so that without running any risks, you can wait for your metabolism to calm down and for the rebound effect to subside. This rebound effect is one of the most common reasons why weight-loss diets do not work.

Length: This depends on how much weight has been lost and can be very easily calculated: 5 days of Consolidation for every pound lost.

Aramis D.—Lost 44 pounds

Keep going; don't look back!

Stabilization forever

We have seen that people who have been overweight know full well that, even after dieting, they will not manage to eat with the moderation and measure that most nutritionists rightly recommend as being the guaranteed way to keep them at the weight they have slimmed down to. This is why it is important to support someone who has just finished his or her Consolidation phase, bearing in mind that his or her personality is that of a person who used to be "fat."

In this fourth phase, the Dukan Diet requires you to eat pure proteins 1 day a week (usually on Thursdays).

Length: For as long as possible, even better, for the rest of your life. By following the few measures in Phase 4, you will be able to eat like everyone else without regaining any weight.

Selen B.—Lost 28 pounds

If you can breathe, you can lose weight on this plan.

A diet that includes lots of water

It is important to drink at least 1½ liters of water per day because once proteins are digested, waste products get into the body in the form of uric acid.

Moreover, if you drink water, this diet works better because although losing weight is about burning calories, it is also about eliminating waste. Just like any other combustion process, the energy burned when you diet produces waste products, and these have to be excreted. Not only does not drinking enough slow down your weight loss, it can also be toxic for your body.

A low-sodium diet

The Dukan Diet makes the body expel water and therefore fights effectively against water retention. Eating food that is too salty will keep the water in your tissues. Remember that 1 liter of water weighs 2 pounds, and it only takes 2 teaspoons of salt for your tissues to store 1 liter of water!

The Dukan Diet's three specific and innovative fundamentals

1. Oat bran

Not all oat brans are of equal value.

There are two types of oat bran:

- **cooking bran** to make desserts, porridge, pancakes, bread, etc.
- **nutritional bran,** whose medicinal benefits are due to the particular way of producing the bran that is based on how the cereal is milled and sifted. Milling involves grinding the bran. Sifting is the process that separates the bran from the oat flour. If the bran is milled too fine, it is much less effective. Likewise, bran that is too coarse will lose its useful surface viscosity. The same goes for the sifting; if the bran is not thoroughly sifted, the oat flour—which is very sugary—will remain in it. The ideal milling is one that produces medium-size particles, i.e., what is technically called M2bis. As for sifting, it is after it has been sifted for a sixth time, B6, that the bran is guaranteed to have a negligible fast carbohydrate content. **The M2bis-B6 index** is awarded when this particular milling and sifting are combined, and it is this **that is responsible for the bran's medicinal properties.**

STAYING ON TRACK

Oat bran is five times richer in the antioxidant beta-glucan than rolled oats. Studies show that beta-glucan helps to lower LDL and supports healthy blood-sugar levels and the immune system! Consuming 2 to 3 tablespoons of oat bran ensures you are getting beta-glucan every day. (Our Oat Bran Cookies are a delicious and healthy way to enjoy these health benefits.)

And what about wheat bran?

Unlike oat bran, **wheat bran** is made up of insoluble fiber, which is of no use whatsoever if you want to lose weight but can be helpful if you become constipated. Its texture and consistency can give some recipes body and density. If you are suffering from constipation, you can add an extra tablespoon of wheat bran to your daily dose of oat bran.

2. Food flavorings

In general, the evolution of the species associates the most appealing smells and flavors with those foods that most contribute to the survival of the animal for which they are intended. This is why the flavor of fats and sugars is so appealing and pleasant: they provide the most energy. Nowadays, we have discovered how to produce flavorings without using the actual food, which means we can enjoy the taste and smell of a food without any of the calories that come with it.

It is easy to see that these food flavorings make losing weight easier. These new tools open up a whole new vista for my diet by making it possible to combine freedom of quantities and freedom of tastes. Unfortunately, many of these flavorings are not yet widely available in supermarkets and for the time being can only be found on the Internet.

STAYING ON TRACK

You likely already know that eating sugar can cause fat storage, hunger, and fatigue, but it also can cause wrinkles and accelerate aging. What foods should you be avoiding? Anything with table sugar, as well as sugars found in processed foods and simple carbs—white bread, pasta, potatoes, rice, corn and corn products, cereals, and snack foods such as chips, popcorn, and pretzels. Consuming natural zero-calorie sweeteners such as luo han from monk fruit or stevia, which are found in many Dukan Diet products, can help you overcome your sweet cravings without contributing to aging and wrinkles.

3. Shirataki noodles

This is a food used in Japanese cooking; Japanese women along with French women share the prize for being the slimmest women on Earth with the longest life spans.

Konjac is like an enormous beet. It has been used in Japan for thousands of years. What makes it so special is the fiber it is composed of, its glucomannan, which means it has much to offer, just like the pectin in apples and the beta-glucans in oat bran. Konjac fiber can absorb up to one hundred times its weight in water, forming an ultraviscous gel that fills up the stomach, trapping fats and sugars. However, what is magical is that this all takes place with practically NO CALORIES. Konjac has virtually no calories but is very filling—which is why this marvelous ingredient caught my interest.

Konjac comes in various forms (blocks, vermicelli, powder, etc.), but the best way for Europeans/Westerners to use Konjac is as noodles or shirataki. They have a very pleasant texture and are slightly chewy but do not taste like anything in particular. However, they do soak up the flavor of the sauce or whatever they are mixed into.

In the Dukan Diet, the most common way of serving shirataki noodles is with a Bolognese sauce made with ground meat and a homemade or store-bought tomato sauce, but this must be sugar-free and fat-free.

In the Attack phase, you can eat shira-

How do you use oat bran in each phase?

- In the Attack phase, 1½ tablespoons per day
- In the Cruise phase, 2 tablespoons per day
- In the Consolidation phase, 2 tablespoons per day
- In the Stabilization phase and for the rest of your life, 3 tablespoons per day

You can buy oat bran to make your own galettes, porridge, and bread. Recently products have appeared that contain oat bran as the only grain, such as oat bran cookies, oat bran bars, and muffins. Always choose organic oat bran and if possible bran with the M2bis-B6 index.

taki noodles by cutting down on the tomato sauce and sticking with the ground meat. In the Cruise phase, all sorts of vegetables can be added to the Konjac, such as diced eggplant and zucchini, strips of sweet bell pepper, etc. In the Consolidation phase, add some parmesan, and in the Stabilization phase you can add whatever you like.

In the fight against weight problems, shirataki noodles offer an unprecedented step forward. Lots of different recipes are available, and ready-made meals have been produced to familiarize people with this food, which is still not widely used or known.

STAYING ON TRACK

Vegetables such as asparagus, beets, broccoli, brussels sprouts, cabbage, carrots, celery, green beans, lettuce, onions, pumpkin, spinach, and tomatoes are high in potassium, which can help with leg cramps and prevent salt cravings.

Questions and answers

Should I ask my doctor to monitor me while I'm on the Dukan Diet?

Losing weight is a serious decision and you should talk to your doctor about what you are planning to do. Why? Because your doctor knows you and you trust him or her. Your doctor will tell you if you really do need to lose weight and will get you to take a few tests—a blood sample—for three reasons:

- **First,** to confirm you don't have a lazy thyroid. Because if you do, you can follow whatever diet you want but without any hope of losing weight.
- **Second,** if you have a serious kidney problem, you'll need to reduce your protein intake and eat more vegetables.
- **Third,** to check whether you have dyslipidemia (too much cholesterol or triglycerides), diabetes, or pre-diabetes—you'll be pleased to see your levels decrease as you diet.

Place your trust in your doctor. Your doctor's help is welcome, reassuring, and invaluable.

Can I use protein bars and powders?

No. There are two reasons for this:

Most of the bars sold in stores are high in carbohydrates, and compared with what is recommended in this diet, their protein content is far too low. Whenever you cannot cook, go for food that is easy to eat, such as cooked chicken or turkey slices and seafood sticks. You can also stock up your fridge with fat-free ricotta and yogurt.

Recently, bars have become available that are compatible with the Dukan Diet, without any added fat or sugar but based exclusively on oat bran. They have been specially created as snacks that are allowed while following the diet.

On their own, protein powders are not allowed in the Dukan Diet since they are artificial, processed products. However, they can be used to increase the protein content of main dishes and desserts.

Only synthetic protein powders contain enough protein, but our program works with real, natural proteins and not with powdered ones. In the Stabilization phase, and only as a stopgap, you may use protein powders such as whey, soy, or brown rice protein.

Arthur J.—Lost 112 pounds

Don't cheat—nothing tastes as good as skinny feels, LOL!

How can I diet and watch my cholesterol?

You just have to be particularly careful with eggs. If your cholesterol is not elevated, you can have one whole egg per day. If your cholesterol level is a little too high, then cook just with egg whites. If this is the case, make your oat bran galette using only the egg white (see the recipe on page 48). Otherwise, eat as many egg whites as you want, but limit yourself to four yolks per week.

I tend to skip meals—will this speed up my diet?

Quite the opposite. You must make sure that you never skip meals—it is completely counterproductive and should be avoided at all costs! If, for example, you skip lunch, the chances are that by 5 p.m. you will be ravenous at a time when, no doubt, you will feel like devouring a bar of chocolate. However, let's imagine that you hold on until dinner. You are then bound to eat more and choose more comforting foods—starchy foods, bread, fatty products, and so on. And your body is going to penalize you too by extracting as much as it can from whatever you feed it with. From what you eat at each meal, the body extracts a reasonable amount from the food. Let's say that it takes 70 to 75 percent. If you skip lunch, not only will you eat more at the next meal, but your body will extract up to 95 percent.

SLIMMING SECRET #2—
CARDAMOM AND CORIANDER

When you lose weight there are two small problems that may bother you: bad breath and constipation—along with its twin sister abdominal bloating. If your breath becomes embarrassing for you, think of cardamom. The simplest thing to do is to infuse it in some green tea. For your abdominal bloating, it's coriander that you need. Use it in everything—in your vinaigrette dressings, in your soups (1 pinch per bowl), and on all your white meats. A secret within the secret: If you are really worried about your breath, peel and crush together some cardamom and coriander. Add this mixture to your normal toothpaste, and use it to brush your teeth and tongue.

Ann A.—Lost 50 pounds

I have to tell you all that the one thing that helped me on the diet is the oat bran. I make so many things out of it now, and I don't miss bread anymore. I love the galettes and all the things I can make with the oat bran!

In a nutshell . . . the Dukan method in twelve key points

1 Effectiveness

I know of nobody who, having followed the diet with motivation and confidence, has not lost weight, attained their True Weight, then consolidated and stabilized it.

2 It works quickly

With the Attack, the diet gets going with lightning speed, maintaining, and even increasing, motivation tenfold.

3 Simplicity

100 foods, 68 proteins (including sugar-free gelatin), 32 vegetables, plus shirataki noodles

4 No hunger

The 100 foods come with the magic words "as much as you want."

5 A clear structure based on four phases

Precise and clear guidance on which to lean. A non-negotiable road map from which it is hard to deviate.

6 Each person has their True Weight

This concept enables every overweight person who is about to start dieting to calculate what their correct weight should be. Your True Weight is an "attainable and maintainable" weight.

7 A natural method

The 100 foods in my diet are fundamentally human. Almost all of these are foods that we have always eaten, the "hunter-gatherers' foods."

8 A stabilization contract

Three simple, concrete measures, prescribed for life.

9 An intuitive program

Learn to lose weight by instinctively understanding the importance of foods according to the order in which they are introduced.

10 The PE concept

"Prescribed exercise" is a radically new way of prescribing the second driving force behind weight loss, just like medication.

11 The method now includes personalization

A weight-loss program stands a much better chance of succeeding if it is personalized. With the Internet, this is now possible (see pages 155–157).

12 The diet now includes online monitoring and coaching

Monitoring, day after day, pound after pound, is finally available on the Internet, where the diet has become interactive through the exchange of morning instructions and the user's evening reports (see pages 155–157).

Attack

The pure proteins phase gets the diet off to a lightning start. Once you are following it, you are in control of a mighty bulldozer that will crush all resistance in its path. So get on board!

What you are aiming
for in Phase 1

Just one instruction to follow: you can eat as much as you want of the foods that are allowed

In the following pages, you will find a list of foods you are allowed to eat (see pages 44 and 45). They are yours, and you can eat as much of them as you want. As for other foods, forget about them for the time being.

Make sure you drink at least 1½ liters of water per day. By drinking this much, you will feel as if there is "something there," and you will also feel full more quickly. You may need to go to the bathroom a lot because your kidneys, not being used to your drinking so much, are forced to open their valves and eliminate. Very soon, you'll seem so much lighter, your face will be thinner and rings will slip off, since your fingers are no longer swollen!

The Attack diet uses "the surprise effect": your body will just have to get used to a new way of eating.

The first day on this Attack diet

This is a day of adjustment and combat. Of course the door is wide open to many categories of common and tasty foods, but it is closed to many others that you are used to eating. To get your diet started, try and choose a day when you can relax and are free to feed yourself as you want. The start of a weekend may be ideal, but you decide, depending on how your week is structured.

During these first three days, you will feel very restricted. To remedy this and stay on course, make sure you fill your fridge with the foods you are allowed. Then you can take full advantage of what this diet offers as, for the first time, you can eat "as much as you want" of foods as dense and prized as beef, veal, fish, and shellfish of every kind (including smoked salmon, canned tuna, seafood sticks (surimi), oysters, and shrimp), as well as scrambled eggs, the endless variety of fat-free dairy products, and low-fat sliced meats—the choice is yours! So on the first day, eat more. Make up for what you cannot eat with the quantity of what you can have.

The second day

During these first two days you might feel a little tired and less inclined to any prolonged effort. Your body has been "taken by surprise" during the Attack phase, and it is burning up calories without counting or resisting, so this is not the right time to put it through an intense workout. During this period, avoid hard physical exercise and extreme sports.

From the third day onward

Your tiredness will go, and it is usually replaced by a sense of euphoria and dynamic energy that are further reinforced by the encouraging message on your scales. Your hunger also disappears. This surprising disappearance is due to ketone bodies being released, the most powerful natural appetite suppressants. It may also be caused by weariness in anyone who is not a great meat-and-fish eater—monotony has a marked effect on appetite. After this third day, raging hunger and cravings for sweet things disappear.

A decisive weight loss

A real psychological turning point and surprise for your metabolism, this Attack phase should enable you to lose, quickly and effectively, as much weight as your body can lose during this short length of time. You will be surprised by it.

The rules for Phase 1

How long?

The Attack phase consists of pure proteins. How long this stage lasts will vary according to your age, how much weight you have to lose, and how many diets you have previously tried. Here are a few ideas to help you set your target clearly and stick to it.

A solution for constipation

Constipation comes about because protein foods contain very little fiber. Buy some oat bran and add it to your yogurt. Most important, drink as much as you are supposed to. In addition to the well-known fact that water makes you urinate, drinking also adds water to your stools. This softens them and makes it much easier for them to pass through the system, which eases digestion.

Your mouth feels dry

Having a dry mouth and bad breath are symptoms that occur with any weight-loss diet and will be a little more noticeable here than they might be with more gradual diets. These symptoms are therefore a sign that you are indeed losing weight, and so you should welcome them as proof of your success. To ease them, you should drink more water and use sugar-free chewing gum.

Rebecca W.—Lost 38 pounds

The first few all-protein days are challenging. But after that, I swear, you will not be starving, the plan will not be hard to stick to, and best of all, I guarantee it will work!

To lose under 10 pounds

You are recommended to avoid an all-too-rapid start—a single day may be enough. This first day, the opening day, has the advantage of providing a complete break with the past that takes your body by surprise, producing an astonishing weight loss that is enough to encourage you to get going with the diet.

To lose under 20 pounds

I would suggest you start with a three-day Attack phase, which will allow you to proceed effortlessly to the alternating proteins (Cruise) phase.

To lose between 20 and 40 pounds

To lose this amount, the Attack phase should last five days. This is the length of time needed to allow the diet to provide the best results without your metabolism developing resistance or your growing weary of it. This is usually how long the Attack phase lasts.

To lose over 40 pounds

With major obesity, when a person wants to lose over 40 pounds, it is possible to carry on with the pure proteins phase for up to seven, and even ten, days. You may also opt for this time period (after talking to your doctor) if you have previously tried lots of diets, as your body is very likely to be stubbornly resistant. In this case, it is absolutely essential that you drink at least 1½ liters of water per day.

How do you keep on course?

- Read, and keep reading, your list of allowed foods very carefully, drawing up a shopping list for the ones you enjoy eating. Don't just rely on this list, but follow the instructions that can be summed up in just a few words: lean meat, fish and shellfish, poultry, lean sliced cooked meats, eggs, tofu, fat-free dairy products, and water.
- Eat as often as you want. The diet allows quantity, so make the most of this!
- Never skip a meal, as this would be a serious mistake. You will eat more at the next meal or, even worse, give in and eat foods you are not allowed. And your body will make you pay dearly for this extra restriction.
- Drink a lot, and drink every time you eat. To get rid of waste properly, you absolutely must drink at least 1½ liters of water per day. Water will also help you feel replete.
- Fill up your fridge! If you should happen to run out of proteins and feel hungry, you are going to binge on some food you are not allowed. Make sure that you shop regularly so you do not have to go without.

Three meals a day

Even if the principle of this diet is based on your being able to eat as much as you want of the foods on the list we give you, nonetheless it is important to stick to a normal eating pattern with three meals. First and foremost, if you skip a meal, your body will "take revenge" at the next meal. You are likely to cave in to foods that are not allowed, and then your body, which by definition dislikes any frustration, will hoard even more from the foods you do give it.

Weigh yourself!

During the Attack phase, keep on weighing yourself because this will keep you in good spirits as, hour by hour, you see your scale veer in the right direction. Your scale is your friend. It will give you encouragement during the Attack and Cruise phases and help you to remain vigilant during the Consolidation and Stabilization phases.

STAYING ON TRACK

Make sure you are eating meals at regular intervals to maintain stable blood-sugar levels.

When will it be difficult?

The first three days may be a tricky time, since your body is going to have to get used to this new way of eating.

You will have to get the better of your hunger, which will fade away from the third day onward. And you are going to feel constipated, but the oat bran will soon sort this out.

You may also find that during the first three days you have an intense longing for sweet things. Hold firm—three days is not the end of the world. If you manage to stay the course, your hunger, as well as compulsive cravings for sugar, will disappear as your diet evolves.

Walk!

Don't forget to walk every day for 20 minutes. This is not just a suggestion or a piece of advice; this is a two-way contract that you have to stick to.

Courtney K.—Lost 85 pounds

Just tell yourself when you are craving something that you can have it later. The diet is not forever!

Pure proteins

What are they?

Of all the foodstuffs we eat, only egg white is made up of virtually pure proteins. However, there are a certain number of foods that come close to the perfection we are seeking, which is why you will find the following proteins (all extremely rich in pure proteins) on the list of foods allowed during this first phase:

- beef (but not rib-eye steak, rib of beef, or any cuts for stewing)
- veal
- poultry (except for duck and goose)
- fish
- shellfish
- eggs
- fat-free dairy products
- vegetarian proteins: tofu, seitan

SLIMMING SECRET #3—

CHOCOLATE

If you have a passion for chocolate, it's because you love the richness and smoothness that defines cocoa. Yet it's in cocoa's powder where its stimulating effects are concentrated. Cocoa has antidepressant properties and contains phenylethylamine—a feel good substance. Cocoa's magnesium provides a soothing and tranquilizing effect. Theobromine and caffeine are compounds in cocoa responsible for its strong sensory and emotional charge. The rest of the cocoa is made up of cocoa butter and sugar—this adds calories and saturated fat. When dieting, buy real low-fat cocoa powder from a health food store and start adding it to yogurt, fat-free milk, and your fat-free cream cheese. Treat yourself and lose weight at the same time!

The law of all or nothing

How effective Phase 1 is will depend entirely on the foods selected. The diet will work with lightning speed provided you eat only from this category of foods. But be careful: if you do not follow this instruction to the letter, your diet will be slowed down, even blocked or ruined. So you must not allow yourself any extras whatsoever. To you a tiny square of chocolate after your grilled meat may appear harmless, but for your body it changes everything. As we have explained earlier, the principle of the diet is based on your body having to digest proteins and nothing else. If you introduce sugars or fats into your day, your protein fasting will be compromised.

Derek C.—Lost 65 pounds

Add a little wheat bran if you get constipated— and lots of water in the beginning.

It is impossible, therefore, to follow this diet halfheartedly. The Dukan Diet obeys the law of all or nothing. If you decide to follow it "a little," its metabolic effectiveness will be put in jeopardy.

On the other hand, if you stick to this single instruction without deviation, your diet will drive your body to:

- burn up calories to digest the proteins;
- digest the protein foods more slowly;
- very quickly draw on its reserves without diminishing either your muscles or your bones;
- eliminate waste and get rid of cellulite;
- fight against edema and water retention; and
- reduce its appetite.

Take heart: this stage does not last very long, so hold on tight and keep going!

An ideal diet to tackle water retention

You can also use the pure proteins phase if at times in your life you feel that you are putting on a pound or two here and there. Two or three days of pure proteins can put your body back on track again. This comment is aimed in particular at those women who feel bloated at the end of their menstrual cycle and at women who, around the age of 50, start noticing their body change even though they are not eating any more than usual. How and why women put on weight happens to be more complex than it is for men and is often linked with water retention. A few days of pure proteins will mean you no longer feel bloated, and this phase in the diet is really good at dealing with the feeling of heavy legs and pudgy fingers, etc. In addition to the results displayed on your scales, you will rediscover your real shape, and your figure will be transformed.

After following your diet, you will be able to enjoy all the beneficial effects of Phase 1 throughout your life thanks to the Protein Thursdays that we will introduce in the Stabilization phase.

Gaining weight in menopause

Obviously, menopause is a very tricky time in a woman's life as far as weight is concerned, but we must not throw in the towel. As soon as the first few pounds start to take hold, it is important to act. If this happens, one Protein Thursday per week or two days every two weeks may be enough to keep you at your ideal weight. As for the other days, avoid drinking too much water, and go easy with the salt to limit water retention. While we are on this subject, stop eating ready-made meals—they alone are responsible for almost 90 percent of the salt we consume!

The 68 foods allowed in Attack

Always have on hand or in your fridge a wide selection from the food categories that are going to become your friends and your best-loved foods. When you are out and about, take them with you, as most protein foods require some preparation and, unlike carbohydrates and fats, do not keep as well and cannot be found as easily as biscuits and chocolate in drawers and cupboards.

Before you eat a food, make sure that it appears on the list on pages 44 and 45. Never be without the foods you need for your diet. To be really sure of what you are doing, keep this list with you during the first week. It is simple and boils down to just a few words: lean meats and organ meats, fish and shellfish, poultry, sliced cooked meats, eggs, fat-free dairy products, and drinks.

How should I cook my meat?

Meats should be prepared without using any fat, butter, oil, or cream, even if it is low-fat. You are advised to grill your meat, but these meats can also be roasted in the oven or on a rotisserie, cooked in foil parcels, or even boiled. How much you cook them is left to each individual's personal preference, but remember that cooking gradually removes the fat from the meat, bringing it closer to the ideal pure protein state that underlies this diet. Go ahead and use spices to avoid monotony.

Lean meats

Beef

All cuts for roasting or grilling are allowed—in particular, steaks, filet, sirloin, roast beef, and other lean cuts.

Ground beef

Uncooked ground beef can be prepared tartare- or carpaccio-style, but without any oil. It can also be mixed with an egg, some herbs, and capers, shaped into meatballs and cooked in the oven.

Ground beef is allowed, but make sure that the fat content does not exceed 10 to 15 percent fat, which is too rich for the Attack period.

Veal

Veal cutlets and roast veal are recommended. Veal chops are allowed as long as all the surrounding fat is cut off.

Rabbit

A source of lean meat that can be eaten roasted or cooked with mustard and fat-free sour cream or ricotta.

Organ meats

You can eat calf's and lamb's tongue as well as liver. Liver contains many vitamins, which are extremely useful during a weight-loss diet. However, it does contain cholesterol, so if you have cholesterol problems, eat liver in moderation.

Fish

There is no restriction or limitation with this family of foods. All fish are allowed, whether they are lean or fatty, white or oily, fresh or frozen, canned in brine or water (not in oil), smoked or dried.

All fatty and oily fish

They are all allowed—in particular, sardines, mackerel, tuna, and salmon.

Smoked fish

Although smoked salmon looks shiny and greasy, it is hardly any fattier than a 90 percent fat-free steak. The same goes for smoked trout, eel, and haddock.

Canned fish

Very handy for quick meals or snacks, canned fish is allowed if it is in water or brine, like tuna and salmon, or mackerel without sauce.

How should I cook my fish?

Fish should be cooked without adding any fat. Sprinkle it with lemon juice and herbs and spices, or bake it in the oven stuffed with herbs and lemon. You can also steam it or, even better, cook it in a foil packet so that you keep in all the cooking juices.

Wild or farmed salmon?

Choose wild Alaskan salmon instead of farmed salmon, since the wild variety is higher in omega-3 fatty acids, which reduce inflammation in the body and support weight loss. Farmed salmon is usually fed grains such as corn, making it higher in omega-6—therefore you are not getting the benefit of eating oily fish when you choose farm-raised salmon.

Seafood sticks (surimi)

Made from extremely lean white fish, seafood sticks are totally allowed. They are very handy and easy to take around with you.

Shellfish

You may eat as much as you want of crayfish, clams, crab, shrimp, lobster, oysters, mussels, scallops, squid, and octopus. They will add a festive touch to your diet.

What should I drink?

All types of water are allowed, especially spring waters that are slightly diuretic, just as long as they do not contain too much sodium. For older people, it is best to drink water with a high calcium and magnesium content. If you do not care much for still water, you may drink carbonated water, as the bubbles and gas have no effect on this diet. However, you should avoid San Pellegrino, for example, which is excellent but contains too much sodium for this diet. If you really must, you can have one glass per day, but no more. Perrier is a better choice.

Poultry

All poultry is allowed, except birds with flat beaks, such as farm-reared ducks and geese. Be careful not to eat any skin, and choose organic poultry, if possible.

Chicken
Of the different parts, the white breast meat is the leanest; then choose the legs and, last, the wings.

Turkey
Acceptable in all forms. Try pan-fried cutlets or a roast drumstick stuffed with garlic.

Low-fat sliced and cooked meats, with any rind cut off

Fine if lean, low-fat, and trimmed of all rind. With cooked meat, go for ham or turkey slices, as they only have a fat content of between 2 and 4 percent. They are handy for quick snack lunches.

You are allowed to drink diet fizzy drinks (Coca-Cola Zero and other diet sodas).

Remember, too, that you can drink sugar-free, fruit-flavored water (Polar Ice, Poland Spring, etc.) which will give you flavors you might be missing. You can also drink tea, herbal teas, and chicory-based drinks.

STAYING ON TRACK

Need to add some calcium to your diet? Canned salmon and sardines with bones, firm tofu, collard greens, turnip greens, dandelion greens, spinach, and kale are great Dukan-friendly sources of this mineral. (Just remember to eat phase-appropriately.)

Eggs

Whole eggs
They can be eaten hard-boiled, soft-boiled, poached, or fried, in an omelet or scrambled in a nonstick frying pan—i.e., without adding any oil or butter. Look for organic or pastured eggs.

Matthew K.—Lost 116 pounds

Take joy in the foods you CAN eat.

Egg white on its own

Eggs are high in cholesterol, and their excessive consumption should be avoided by anyone with an unusually high cholesterol level. You are recommended to eat only three or four egg yolks a week, whereas the white, a pure protein par excellence, may be eaten without any restriction. If this is the case, it may also be a good idea to make your omelets and scrambled eggs using one yolk to two whites.

Vegetarian proteins

For those who prefer vegetarian food, these proteins offer more choices. The vegetarian proteins listed here are made from soy and wheat:

- **Tofu** can be firm tofu to be used in your starters, soups, and main course recipes or silken tofu, ideal for mousse, oat bran quiches, and even for whisking into light sauces.

Sweeteners

Sugar is not allowed but sweeteners are. Here are the most common ones:

- **aspartame,** which has been used for more than twenty years by over a billion people across the world, without to date any incident being reported. If heated to a high temperature, powdered aspartame loses some of its ability to sweeten.
- **stevia,** best used for dishes that are cold or slightly heated; it particularly suits fruity recipes, as it has a faint taste of licorice.
- Other sweeteners will vary depending on the country. In France, the health authorities allow the use of cyclamate, saccharin, and sucralose. Cyclamate is banned in the United States. Your choice of sweetener must be based on what it is to be used for: saccharin is best used to sweeten drinks, and sucralose (**Splenda**) is best in cold or baked desserts or if cooking at a high temperature.

It is a good idea to use a wide range of different sweeteners so that you avoid using a single product repeatedly. We recommend the natural sweetener stevia.

- **Seitan or "vegetable meat"** is just like tofu, but it is made from wheat proteins. Perfect for stews, stuffings, and kebabs.

Fat-free dairy products

Fat-free plain dairy products
Yogurt, sour cream, cottage cheese, ricotta, cream cheese—you can eat as much as you want of them.

Fat-free, sugar-free flavored dairy products (vanilla, coconut, lemon, and so on)
You can eat them as much as you want.

Fat-free dairy products with fruit, but sugar-free
In Phase 1, they are tolerated, but it would be better to avoid them. Ideally, in Attack, you will not eat them, but one can be tolerated.

Fat-free milk
Fresh or powdered, it is allowed. Fat-free milk can also be used to make sauces, creams, custards, and in a range of other dishes.

STAYING ON TRACK

Try not to bargain with yourself for your favorite snack from before you started the diet. Even if you find a sugar-free/fat-free alternative, chances are it is completely fake and full of unnecessary chemicals and substitutes. And it won't even taste like the real thing! It is just a gateway to craving the real thing.

Drinks

It is absolutely vital you drink at least 1½ liters of liquid per day during your diet. This is not a recommendation, but a requirement. The quantity of liquid is non-negotiable for two reasons:

- Once the body digests the proteins, they release a great amount of waste products into your body in the form of urea. To get rid of these waste products, it is absolutely vital that you drink enough.
- Throughout your diet, your body will get rid of stored fat, and water will help your body with this. By drinking copiously, you will be draining it thoroughly.

Seasoning and spices

Thyme, garlic, parsley, onion, shallots, chives, and so on, as well as all spices, are not only allowed but are heartily recommended. By using them, you can enhance the flavor of the dishes you eat so the food leaves you feeling replete and satisfied afterward.

Even if you are doing everything you should, you will stop losing weight if you do not drink enough. Instead of being flushed out, the waste produced from burning up your fat will accumulate.

Seasonings and condiments

You will find the exhaustive list of the condiments you are allowed on page 45.

Salt

Salt is allowed but must be eaten in moderation, especially if you suffer from water retention. If you are experiencing menopause or pre-menopause, avoid salt, or opt instead for reduced-sodium salts. Choose Celtic or Himalayan sea salt.

Oil

Although some oils, such as olive oil, are rightly reputed as being good for the heart and arteries, they are nonetheless oils and pure fats and so have no place in this pure protein diet. You can, however, use up to a teaspoon for a vinaigrette mixture for several people, or ⅛ of a teaspoon of oil to grease a pan.

Vinegar

Vinegar is very much a feature of this diet. Choose strong-tasting vinegars such as balsamic, apple cider, and sherry vinegar, but avoid the cheapest ones as some inexpensive balsamic vinegars contain caramel and therefore lots of sugar.

Lemon juice

This can be used to flavor fish and shellfish, but it cannot be consumed as a lemon juice drink or lemonade, even without sugar, because then the lemon is no longer a condiment but a fruit. It is sour to be sure, but nevertheless a source of sugar and incompatible with pure proteins.

Rachel K.—Lost 29 pounds

Set mini goals.

Mustard

Mustard must be eaten in moderation during this Attack phase. There are salt-free mustards if you suffer from water retention.

Pickles and pickled onions

They are allowed if used as condiments, but they cease being part of a pure protein diet if used in such quantities that they have to be considered vegetables.

Ordinary ketchup

This is not allowed as it is both very salty and very sweet. However, there are sugar-free diet ketchups that may be used in moderation.

What can you eat in Phase 1?

Meat (choose grass-fed meat when possible)

Allowed

Beef tenderloin, filet mignon, flank, sirloin, London broil
Buffalo
Extra-lean ham
Extra-lean kosher beef hot dogs
Ground beef (at least 90% lean)
Pork tenderloin, pork loin roast, lean center-cut pork chops
Rabbit
Veal chops and cutlets
Venison

Not allowed

Lamb
Pork ribs
Rib of beef
Rib-eye steak

Organ meats

Allowed

Calf's liver
Kidney
Tongue (calf's, lamb's, and beef tip)

Not allowed

Beef tongue (the fatty bottom part)
Ox tongue

Cooked meats

Allowed

Bresaola (air-dried/wind-dried beef)
Fat-free turkey and chicken sausage
Lean deli slices of roast beef
Low-fat deli slices of chicken or turkey
Reduced-fat bacon, soy bacon

Not allowed

Cured ham
Smoked ham

Fish

Allowed

Arctic char
Catfish
Cod
Fish roe (cod, herring, salmon)
Flounder
Grouper
Haddock
Halibut and smoked halibut
Herring
Mackerel
Mahi-mahi
Monkfish
Orange roughy
Perch
Red snapper
Salmon and smoked salmon
Sardines
Sea bass
Shark
Sole
Surimi
Swordfish
Tilapia
Trout
Tuna, fresh or canned in water

Not allowed

Mackerel in sauce
Sardines or tuna in oil

Shellfish

Allowed

Clams
Crab
Crawfish, crayfish
Lobster
Mussels
Octopus
Oysters
Scallops
Shrimp
Squid

Not allowed

None

Poultry (choose organic when possible)

Allowed

Chicken
Chicken liver
Cornish hen
Ostrich steak
Quail
Turkey
Wild duck

Not allowed

Goose

Oat and wheat bran
Allowed
1½ tablespoons oat bran per day
1 tablespoon wheat bran (optional)
Not allowed
None

Eggs (choose organic or pastured eggs when possible)
Allowed
Chicken, quail, and duck eggs
Not allowed
None

Dairy products
Allowed
Fat-free cottage cheese
Fat-free cream cheese
Fat-free milk
Fat-free plain Greek-style yogurt, unsweetened or artificially sweetened
Fat-free ricotta
Fat-free sour cream
Not allowed
Cheese
Whole milk dairy products

Vegetarian proteins
Allowed
Seitan (only for vegetarians)
Soy foods and veggie burgers (only for vegetarians)
Tempeh (only for vegetarians)
Tofu
And
Shiritaki noodles and rice

Condiments
Allowed
Baking powder
Basil
Cardamom
Chervil
Chili powder
Chives
Cinnamon
Cloves
Coriander
Cumin
Garlic
Gelatin
Ginger
Harissa or hot sauce
Horseradish
Lemons and limes (except in drinks)
Lemongrass
Lemon, lime, and orange zest
Low-sodium stock cubes and broths
Mint
Mustard
Nutmeg
Oat bran
Onions/shallots/dried onion
Orange-flower water
Paprika
Parsley
Pepper
Pickles/cornichons/pickled onions
Rosemary
Saffron
Salt
Seaweed
Soy sauce (low sodium)
Star anise
Sugar-free food flavorings
Sugar-free teriyaki sauce
Sweeteners
Tarragon
Thyme
Turmeric
Vanilla (pods, flavoring, and sugar-free powder)
Vinegars
Tolerated
Dukan mayonnaise
Dukan vinaigrette
Goji berries (1 tablespoon)
Sugar-free ketchup (1 tablespoon)
Tomato purée (for cooking) (1 tablespoon)
Not allowed
Butter
Chocolate
Dried fruit
Edamame
Ketchup
Mayonnaise
Nuts
Oils (except for up to 1 teaspoon for a vinaigrette or ⅛ teaspoon to grease a pan)
Olives
Sour cream
Stock cubes (except for low-fat or low-salt)
Sugar

Breakfast

What can you eat for breakfast in Phase 1?

You may choose what you want from this list and create a breakfast menu to suit your tastes.

Drinks

Chicory coffee alternatives
Coffee
Fat-free milk
Tea/herbal teas

Dairy Products

Fat-free cottage cheese
Fat-free cream cheese
Fat-free ricotta
Fat-free yogurt

Crêpes

Oat bran galette (1½ tablespoons oat
  bran maximum; see page 48)

Meat and Eggs

Cooked chicken (without any fat or
  rind)
Cooked ham (without any fat or rind)
Cooked turkey (without any fat or
  rind)
Omelet
Reduced-fat or soy bacon
Scrambled, fried, poached, or soft-
  boiled eggs (with cooked chicken
  breast tenders for dipping)

If you cannot eat anything when you wake up

You must on no account skip this meal. Have a hot drink, wait an hour, and then have breakfast.

How can I go without bread?

You will have realized that for breakfast there is no deviation from the list of allowed foods, which is why you will not see any toast, rolls, muffins, bagels, etc., on your menus. However, there are plenty of other foods that you can fill yourself up with, since you may eat your fill of fat-free dairy products (natural or with stevia) or tuck a slice of lean chicken into a soft-boiled egg. You will feel as if you have enjoyed a very full breakfast—a little like having a full brunch every morning!

Matthew S.—Lost 86 pounds

If you can make it past 1 month there is no looking back. If I can do it, anyone can do it.

Moreover, this menu will be more energizing and balanced than a traditional breakfast of toast, muffins, bagels, or chocolatey cereals.

STAYING ON TRACK

Banish boredom—many dieters overeat not because they're hungry but because they're bored. Next time you feel that way, don't head for the pantry, head for the door and get out of the house—catch up on window shopping, or drop in on a friend and suggest going for a walk.

Alatha G.—Lost 47 pounds

The scale—once an enemy—make it your best friend! Also, always make sure you have plenty of food ready; you are less likely to cheat if you open the fridge and your yummy yogurt is staring at you. I also always keep a bunch of hard-boiled eggs in the fridge for a quick snack!

The oat bran galette

For some of my patients, mornings are the time of day when they most miss having the taste of bread. Others also complain about constipation. To get around these inconveniences and for die-hard bread fans, hearty eaters, and people with constipation, I devised a galette recipe that can be included in the protein diet.

This came about when my daughter wanted to follow my diet. She used to feel ravenous all morning and had trouble keeping going until lunch. So she asked me what she could eat in the morning to "fill" herself up more. I searched through my cupboards and improvised an oat bran galette with some oat bran I had brought back from America, and she thought it was

Oat bran galette recipe

2 tablespoons oat bran*
1 whole egg or just the white
1½ teaspoon fat-free plain Greek yogurt
⅛ teaspoon stevia or a little salt (according to taste)

Combine the oat bran and the egg white or whole egg (depending on your appetite and cholesterol level) with the yogurt and the sweetener or salt.

Mix together thoroughly, then cook the galette in a nonstick frying pan without any fat (if the galette sticks to your pan, you can wipe a drop of oil over the surface using a paper towel).

If you are suffering from constipation, you can also add 1 teaspoon of wheat bran per day.

*From the Cruise phase onward. In the Attack phase, use only 1½ tablespoons oat bran.

excellent and nutritious. I fine-tuned the recipe, and now oat bran is used systematically in my method. This galette is packed with soluble fiber, and many recent studies have proved that by soaking up water, this soluble fiber forms a gel in the digestive tract. Nutrients get trapped in it, and a few calories get taken away with this gel into the stools.

Sam K.—Lost 40 pounds

Find some favorite foods to fall back on when you are hungry or want to munch on something.

With the help and creativity of the whole Dukan Diet community, new recipes have been developed offering plenty of choice: Dukan muffins, bread, pies, pancakes, desserts, and pastries . . . and certain products such as cookies and bars are now available online.

Make the most of your morning "fat-burning" opportunity

When your body has not been fed, it digs into its fat cells to find some energy. This happens in the mornings when your stomach is empty. This process is called "lipolysis," and it often starts at night once your sugar reserves are used up. As soon as you get more energy by eating breakfast, it stops. Two ideas for making more of this natural "fat-burning" phase are:

- Since your body will go straight for its fat reserves, if you are not too tired, do some exercise as soon as you wake up and before you have any breakfast.
- Follow the breakfast instructions for Phase 1 to the letter and have a hot drink and proteins. These will not halt the fat-burning process, so you will be able to benefit from breakfast throughout the day.

SLIMMING SECRET #4—
GREEN TEA FOR A PLATEAU

If you are following the diet exactly yet your weight is stagnating, don't worry—this happens frequently to dieters. I don't know of anyone who has lost 20 pounds without having experienced at least one plateau, which generally lasts about a week. I call this a "pause." In this situation there are lots of things you can do. First, make sure that it's not due to water retention related to peri-menopause or because a period is imminent. Then, if it's neither of these, I like to suggest green tea. For three days, don't drink any more water, only drink green tea (decaffeinated, if you're caffeine sensitive) throughout the morning, at lunch, at tea time, and in the evening. Cold, hot, or with ice, however you like it, just as long as it's nonstop green tea. If you do this and keep up with the diet (as well as at least a minimum of physical exercise) you stand every chance of breaking through this plateau.

Lunch

What can you eat for lunch in Phase 1?

You can devise your starters, main dishes, and desserts based around the 68 protein foods listed on pages 44 and 45. You will also find on pages 56–59 some menu ideas for a whole week. Drink lots of water at mealtimes. You could have green tea or sparkling water, too. Soft drinks with artificial sweeteners are also allowed. Try using herbs and spices to add variety to what you eat, and also take care with the presentation—nicely presented food is always more appetizing. To season your meat and eggs, refer to page 45. If you do not have time to prepare a sauce, you can easily add some vinegar, pepper, herbs, or spices.

Avoid common errors that can slow down your diet and trigger water retention. Cut down on salt and mustard too.

Drinks

Green tea
Soft drinks with artificial sweeteners
Still or sparkling water or flavored,
  sweetened

Starters

Canned mackerel without the sauce
Chicken breast
Crab
Fat-free chicken or turkey sausage
Hard-boiled egg
Seafood sticks (surimi)
Shrimp
Smoked salmon

Main Courses

Grilled chicken
Hamburger
Roast beef
Roast veal
Scrambled eggs, etc.
Steamed fish
Turkey burger
Wild Alaskan salmon

Accompaniment

Cooked shirataki noodles (with light
  Bolognese sauce, etc.)

Desserts

Egg-based desserts
Fat-free cottage cheese
Fat-free ricotta
Fat-free yogurt, flavored and
  sugar-free
Oat bran galette (if you did not eat
  one for breakfast)

Of course you can allow yourself a snack as soon as you start to feel hungry, provided it is on the list of foods you are allowed.

Here are a few ideas for handy snacks that you can easily carry around with you:

- seafood sticks (surimi)
- hard-boiled eggs
- fat-free yogurt
- sliced ham, turkey, or chicken (without any fat or rind)
- tea or coffee (without sugar or with sweetener)

Sticking to your mealtime routine

It is important that you keep to a routine with your meals, because otherwise after a few days you will end up feeling frustrated. Sitting down at the table to enjoy a hot meal is both convivial and comforting. Of course, for the time being, your meals are made up of protein foods only, but you will discover that it is possible to devise tasty menus using just proteins.

With the menus you create, based on what you enjoy eating, try and make sure you have a separate starter, main course, and dessert. Feel free to adjust your meals to match your appetite. For example, if you are stretched for time or never very hungry in the morning, then you can enjoy the oat bran galette as your lunchtime dessert.

STAYING ON TRACK

Luo han is a fruit that grows in China and has been used both as a sweetener and for its medicinal properties for hundreds of years. It is said to be 300 times sweeter than sugar, so very little is typically needed to satisfy even the biggest sweet tooth. In the amounts it is typically used, it is considered to be essentially calorie-free with a negligible glycemic index and load.

Dinner

What can you eat for dinner in Phase 1?

More than any other meal (especially if you begin your diet in winter), your dinner must include a hot dish, as this will fill you up and you will feel as if you have eaten a proper meal. You are allowed to eat the same foods as for lunch, and you must structure your meal in the same way with a starter, main course, and dessert. As a nice way to end your meal, you can make yourself an herbal tea or some chicory coffee.

Drinks

Chicory coffee alternatives
Herbal teas
Still or sparkling water or flavored, sweetened

Starters

Canned mackerel without the sauce
Chicken breast
Crab
Hard-boiled egg
Lean cooked meat (without any fat or rind)
Seafood sticks (surimi)
Shrimp
Smoked salmon

Main Courses

Grilled chicken
Roast beef
Roast veal
Scrambled eggs, etc.
Steak tartare or chopped steak
Steamed fish
Turkey burger
Wild Alaskan salmon

Accompaniment

Cooked shirataki noodles (with light Bolognese sauce, etc.)

Desserts

Egg-based desserts
Fat-free cottage cheese
Fat-free ricotta
Fat-free yogurt, flavored and sugar-free
Oat bran galette (if you did not eat one for breakfast)

For a delicious frozen treat, add stevia and cocoa powder to your Greek yogurt, mix well, then freeze.

Mindy B.—Lost 72 pounds

My go-to snacks are nonfat Greek yogurt, tuna, or smoked salmon, depending on my desire. You are less likely to cheat if you are full. And if you select food choices similar enough to your cravings, you can get past them without feeling deprived. A dash of cinnamon really zips up yogurt!

Don't give in!

Dinnertime is often a tricky time. Do you come home feeling tired? Do you have to cook for the children? Are you someone who needs something to nibble on while cooking dinner? Become aware of your own habits. If you know that dinnertime is the most difficult time of the day, then here is a tip to get through it: make yourself an oat bran galette and nibble on it while you cook. However, if you do this, you cannot have a galette at any other time of the day.

Andrea C.—Lost 55 pounds

This diet works differently for everyone. Don't compare yourself and your progress to others. If you go off track, get right back on as soon as possible. The longer you stray the harder it is to get back on. Trust the process and see it through to the end!

No doubt you are going to have to sit down and eat with your family, deliberately avoiding eating foods you are not allowed while watching your children dig into their pasta with relish. To resist temptation, go ahead and treat yourself to a snack before the meal. Avoid sitting down to eat feeling famished, as this is bound to jeopardize your diet. Next, try and cook food for the rest of the family that you yourself are not especially keen on. Not that fond of rice? Then cook rice, and you will find it easier not to give in and have some. Do not tempt fate—if you cannot resist bread and cheese, then don't give it to everyone else. Lastly, make absolutely sure that you include some parts of your diet in what everyone else eats, such as chicken or fish for the main course or fat-free ricotta for dessert. Then you will feel as if you are eating with your family, even if you are not allowed some foods.

Look after yourself

So that you allow your body time to digest your last meal, avoid eating too late, and you will sleep better for it.

Even if you are eating on your own, make yourself comfortable, get out a pretty tablecloth, and set the table nicely for your spread—you should feel as if you are dining as normal. Make things cozy for yourself! Also, take your time over your meals. After you have been eating for 20 minutes, the feeling of hunger disappears. If you wolf your dinner down, you will leave the table with your stomach still feeling empty.

Patsy N.—Lost 67 pounds

Give the Attack phase a chance. Instant motivation!

Some Sample Menus for Phase 1 (Attack)

	Monday	Tuesday	Wednesday
Breakfast	Hot drink Fat-free cottage cheese 1 oat bran galette (page 48)	Hot drink Fat-free plain Greek yogurt 1 oat bran galette	Hot drink Fat-free plain Greek yogurt Egg white omelet
Lunch	Roast beef rolls with fat-free cream cheese Shirataki noodles Bolognese (without tomato sauce) Fat-free plain Greek yogurt	Shrimp with low-sodium soy sauce Saffron cod Fat-free ricotta cheese	Cooked chicken breast (without the skin) Herbed meatballs with shirataki noodles and low-sodium soy sauce Muesli ice cream (page 211)
Snack	Fat-free ricotta Can of tuna	Tea or coffee without sugar Fat-free cottage cheese with cinnamon	1 hard-boiled egg 1 oat bran galette
Dinner	Shrimp Chicken strips with apple cider vinegar Poached egg whites in milk	(Oil-free) tuna rillettes with Dukan mayonnaise Chicken cutlets deglazed with balsamic vinegar Homemade vanilla egg custard	Smoked salmon rolls with fat-free cream cheese, garlic, and herbs Sautéed paprika veal cutlet Fat-free ricotta with cinnamon and stevia

Thursday	Friday	Saturday	Sunday
Hot drink	Hot drink	Hot drink	Hot drink
Fat-free plain Greek yogurt	Fat-free cottage cheese	Fat-free plain Greek yogurt	Fat-free cottage cheese
1 oat bran galette	2 slices cooked ham (without fat or rind)	2 slices low-sodium chicken breast	1 soft-boiled egg with chicken breast tenders
Smoked salmon with scrambled eggs (page 160)	Salmon mousse	Canned tuna mixed with fat-free cream cheese	Chicken broth
Grilled bass with herbs	Strips of squid and shirataki noodles with chopped parsley, shallot, and garlic	Turkey cutlet with curry yogurt sauce	Spicy omelet with fresh mint (page 190)
Mint tea sorbet	Vanilla floating island	Lemon mousse	Coffee granita with cinnamon
Surimi sticks	Can of sardines	Fat-free cottage cheese	Tea or coffee without sugar
1 oat bran muffin	Porridge (made with 1½ tablespoons oat bran)		
Steamed mackerel with herbs	Grilled chicken breast tenders	Tuna fish balls with herbs	Smoked salmon parcels filled with fat-free cottage cheese and chives
Oven-baked Mediterranean shrimp with herbes de provence	Pan-fried curried tofu	Oven-baked salmon steak	Beef kebabs
Sugar-free Jell-O	Fat-free ricotta with lemon extract and stevia	Fat-free plain Greek yogurt with lemon extract and stevia	Sugar-free Jell-O

Don't forget your 1½ tablespoons of oat bran, every day.

The On-the-Go Menu that follows calls for Dukan Diet products at times, but they are not the only options available—you may use other brands provided that all the ingredients are Dukan-friendly. Just make sure to look for nitrite-free, sugar-free turkey jerky and low-sodium, sugar-free marinara or tomato sauce. Whenever Dukan Diet bars or cookies are specified, you may substitute with regular oat bran.

Attack Phase: On-the-Go Menu

	Monday	Tuesday	Wednesday
Breakfast	Coffee or tea 1½ tbsp. oat bran in 1 container fat-free Greek yogurt	Coffee or tea Low-fat slices turkey with fat-free cream cheese	Coffee or tea 2 hard-boiled eggs 1 container fat-free Greek yogurt
Lunch	Grilled halibut and a side of shrimp	Can of sardines 1 container fat-free Greek yogurt	Sashimi platter (3 pieces salmon, 3 pieces mackerel, 3 pieces scallops)
Snack	Dukan Turkey Jerky	1½ tbsp. oat bran hot cereal	1½ tbsp. oat bran hot cereal
Dinner	Grilled wild salmon with Dukan Diet Shirataki Noodles	Grilled chicken Deviled eggs	Ground turkey with Dukan Diet Shirataki Noodles

*You may add an additional snack between breakfast and lunch if you are hungry.

Angela L.—Lost 62 Pounds

The good things in life are hard and also very worth it.

Thursday	Friday	Saturday	Sunday
Coffee or tea 1½ tbsp. oat bran in 1 container fat-free Greek yogurt	Coffee or tea 2 hard-boiled eggs	Coffee or tea Omelet stuffed with smoked salmon	Coffee or tea Scrambled eggs with low-fat ham
Can of salmon over Dukan Diet Shirataki Rice, herbs to taste	Grilled tofu 1 container fat-free Greek yogurt	Grilled chicken and 2 hard-boiled eggs	Can of tuna over Dukan Diet Shirataki Noodles, herbs to taste
Dukan Turkey Jerky	1½ tbsp. oat bran hot cereal	1½ tbsp. oat bran hot cereal	1½ tbsp. oat bran hot cereal
Grilled mahi-mahi with Dukan Diet Shirataki Rice	Grilled steak and shrimp	Ground beef with Dukan Diet Shirataki Noodles	Sashimi platter (3 pieces tuna, 3 pieces salmon, 3 pieces yellowtail) Dukan Diet Shirataki Rice

Fitting your diet into your daily life (Phase 1)

Eating with your family

You will be faced with many temptations, especially if you have children. So that you do not succumb, particularly in the Attack phase, you may well decide to feed the children separately and then get your own meal afterward. To make it simpler, you could cook the proteins on their own (chicken in one dish, vegetables in another) so that you can select the food that suits you without disrupting your normal mealtime pattern. Make sure you increase the quantities of meat and keep serving yourself as much as you need so that you keep up with everyone else. This will also avoid your children asking questions, as they might not understand why your plate is half empty. Prepare some "mix-and-match" menus in advance that you can adapt. If, for example, your children love soft-boiled eggs, have an egg for yourself. You can dip turkey strips into your yolk while your children eat bread.

STAYING ON TRACK

Prepare all your Dukan-friendly foods on Sunday—that way you'll be set for the week and you won't be tempted to cheat.

Cocktail hour

If you are having cocktails at home, you can prepare snacks that you can nibble away at without bending your diet rules, such as shrimp cocktail, seafood sticks (surimi), and cubes of cooked turkey. Also, make sure that you have some sparkling water or diet soda so you can quench your thirst without being tempted by any alcohol or fruit juice. Replenish your glass yourself, and never let it get completely empty. This way you will deter any polite guests, thinking they are being nice to you, from pouring you a little champagne or wine!

If you are invited to a friend's home, the situation is not as easily managed, but it is not insurmountable. Before you leave home, fill yourself up with a suitable snack. Since vegetables are not allowed in the Attack phase, it is possible that you will not be able to eat any of the snacks available. If this is the case, ask for a big glass of sparkling water and hold it all the time, as this will give you an excuse not to take any of the dishes the other guests are handing around.

Maxine F.—Lost 50 pounds

Don't worry about eating out or special occasions and holidays. No one cares what's on your plate.

At the restaurant

Here is a situation where the protein diet is easy to follow. You can start with an egg dish, some smoked salmon, or even a seafood platter. You then have a wide choice for your main course: some grilled sirloin, a veal chop, fish, or poultry. If the food takes some time to arrive, take care not to start nibbling food you are not allowed. If you feel that hunger might gnaw away at your stomach if you have to wait too long for your food, then eat something before you go out to the restaurant, such as a boiled egg or seafood sticks.

For the cheese-lover or dessert fan, the difficulty comes after the main course when you risk being carried along by the other guests. Here the best defense strategy is to ask for a coffee, and then you can order more if the conversation keeps going. Otherwise, keep a fat-free plain or flavored, sugar-free yogurt in your car or office—it will let you finish off your meal with the taste of a fresh, creamy dessert.

Questions and answers

When I am on the diet, should I take vitamins?

If the diet does not last long, taking vitamins is optional. However, if the diet is likely to stretch out over a long period, you should add a daily dose of multivitamin supplements, but avoid high doses and taking lots of different pills, as they build up and can end up being toxic. You would do better to have a slice of calf's liver twice a week and 1 tablespoon of brewer's yeast every morning. As soon as you are allowed vegetables, you can make yourself mixed salads with plenty of lettuce, peppers, tomatoes, carrots, and chicory.

STAYING ON TRACK

Tomatoes are a great source of lycopene. Eating foods rich in lycopene is great for your brain and your beauty as it can protect your skin from the sun's harmful rays. Lycopene acts like an internal sunscreen. Eating cooked tomatoes with a small amount of good fat, such as extra-virgin olive oil, increases the absorption of lycopene.

Can I chew sugar-free chewing gum to take the edge off my hunger?

Chewing gum can prove very useful during a diet for snackers who are used to having something to chew in their mouth. To my mind, chewing gum is an excellent help in fighting weight problems. As you finish your last mouthful at dinner, go ahead and chew some chewing gum, as it will stop you from "raiding" your cupboards.

Should I drink at mealtimes?

Failing to drink while you eat quite simply means that you run the risk of forgetting to drink. What is more, drinking while you eat increases the volume in your stomach, making you feel replete and satisfied. Lastly, water dilutes food, slows down its absorption, and makes you feel full for longer. So yes, drink at mealtimes!

I have trouble drinking a lot—what can I do?

Does drinking 1½ liters of water a day seem too much to you? Don't forget to include any tea, coffee, or other infusion or herbal drink that you have. You will soon see that it is very easy to reach the minimum required. Also, remember to try sugar-free or fruit-flavored waters and the other drinks you are allowed as an appetite suppressant so that you feel fuller.

Can I do any sport in the Attack phase?

Only walking is allowed.

If you have a lot of weight to lose, it is preferable in the Attack phase, but also in the Cruise phase, not to expose the heart, circulation, and hip, knee, and vertebrae joints to any excessive effort.

If you are over 55, build up your exercise routine gradually, taking into consideration how overweight you are at the outset as well as the extra load this puts on your body.

During the Attack phase, you are likely to lose weight at an astonishing speed, and if combined with overexercising, this may tire you out and lessen the feeling of well-being that fuels your motivation both physically and mentally. Despite this, one form of exercise is almost always possible, and that is walking. To my mind, walking is by far the best possible exercise, and it's the simplest too. It's natural and easy, and you can go for a walk anywhere, at any time of the day, no matter what you weigh, without any special gear (you can even walk in heels) and without breaking into a sweat or injuring yourself. It costs nothing, but you'll reap a handsome reward.

Taste the foods listed, and try them all! During the first few days, you will tend to go for the foods you already know. But being on this diet is also an opportunity to be adventurous and discover new flavors. Visit a butcher or a fish market, and try fish that frozen food manufacturers do not sell or meats that you don't find in the supermarket.

Ashley P.—Lost 80 pounds

Just try it. Get creative with your ingredients. You'd be surprised that you can cook your favorite foods, only in a healthy way.

Phase 1 summary

It's over—you have finished Phase 1! Now it is time to take stock of how you feel and what you have lost.

You have lost a lot and very quickly

Since the Attack phase works at lightning speed, it is quite possible to lose 4 to 6 pounds in five days. However, someone who is obese will lose pounds more quickly at the start than a person who is already fairly slim and just wants to get his or her figure trim for the summer holidays. Obese dieters can lose up to around 10 pounds in five days.

STAYING ON TRACK

If you rarely cook your own meals and tend to eat out a lot at restaurants, hidden calories and excess sodium can add up quickly! Some restaurants add flour to their omelets, for example, or add butter and oil to grilled proteins. Make sure to ask for your proteins to be cooked bone dry (no salt, oil, butter, etc.).

You haven't lost weight as quickly as you had imagined

First of all, menstrual periods for most women are a time of high water retention. If this is true for you, drink a little less, and use as little salt as possible. You will lose what you had expected a few days after the start of your period.

If this has nothing to do with periods, then take a closer look at your diet. Did you follow it absolutely to the letter?

The other possibility is that you are a more difficult case. Perhaps you have already tried lots of different diets, you have a strong genetic predisposition to putting on weight, you are experiencing premenopause with a hormonal imbalance, or you may even be taking antidepressants or cortisone?

Tiredness connected with salt and water

Salt has an effect on blood pressure. If you don't have any salt in your food, you lower your blood pressure.

Too much water (if you drink more than 2 liters a day) has the same effect. Water cleanses the blood and brings down blood pressure. When these are combined, it can cause the worst scenario. Try not to drink too much in the evenings. This will allow you to avoid getting up throughout the night, as interrupted sleep will make you tired.

If the tiredness does not go away, get your doctor to check your blood pressure, and let your doctor know that following this diet, as you are, does not usually make the dieter tired.

You have been troubled by constipation

Proteins contain only very few waste products, and not having fats reduces lubrication in the digestive tract. Drink a little more, and go for water that is low in sodium.

You felt a little tired

Do you think the diet has made you feel tired? You were not tired before starting it?

If this is the case, this is quite uncommon, but it is possible. It may be that you are not eating enough. Don't forget that there Is no restriction on quantity. Meat is the best natural fatigue-buster, especially red meat, such as lean cuts of grass-fed beef.

STAYING ON TRACK

Hidden sources of sodium in your condiments (such as mustard, hot sauce, or soy sauce) or proteins (deli meats and smoked salmon) can cause you to retain up to 5 pounds of water! Keep your intake of high-sodium foods to a minimum, especially if you are salt sensitive.

The Attack phase in a nutshell

You can eat 68 high-protein foods and nothing else.
This phase can last between one and seven days. Focus on the foods you are allowed and forget about all other food categories.

You can eat as much as you want of these proteins.

You must drink at least 1½ liters of water each day.
This is not a piece of advice, but an obligation.
For the diet to work, it is essential you drink copious amounts.

The nine food categories you are allowed:
- lean meats, such as veal, rabbit, and beef
- some organ meats
- all fish
- all shellfish
- poultry without the skin (but no duck or goose)
- lean sliced deli meats
- eggs
- fat-free dairy products
- vegetarian proteins (tofu, seitan)

To season your food you can use:
- vinegar
- herbs
- spices
- drops of lemon juice
- a little sea salt
- mustard in moderation

To maximize pleasure, quantities are not restricted at all.
So that you feel good, do not limit quantities, but do vary your menus.

During the few Attack days, avoid all lapses.
This brief phase does not last long and is meant to take your body by surprise, so follow the instructions scrupulously.

You can have 1½ tablespoons of oat bran a day, especially in galettes. You can have as much shirataki noodles as you want.

Cruise

**Go from 68 to 100 as-much-as-you-want foods
until you get down to the weight you want.**

What you are aiming
for in Phase 2

Losing weight regularly

After three to five days in the Attack phase, you'll notice that the lack of vegetables and salad in your diet is starting to make itself felt. So you will have no trouble getting into this second phase, in which you alternate days of pure proteins with days of proteins + vegetables. It will last until you reach your True Weight.

Losing weight over the long haul

No doubt, you will notice that your weight loss slows down in this alternating phase. This is quite normal, as your body has to adjust itself to this new phase so that it can get into the diet over the long term. Don't worry, the weight loss from burning up fats is still continuing, and although somewhat camouflaged by the return of water, it is nonetheless carrying on all the while.

As for how long this phase should last, this all depends on how many pounds you want to lose. It will last until you reach the weight you want to get down to.

Becky N.—Lost 50 pounds

Tell your friends what you are doing and let them support you!

Losing weight more steadily

If you have over 40 pounds to lose, experience shows that, on average, you'll settle down to losing around a couple of pounds a week. Of course, during Phase 1 you lost a lot more, which is why within the space of a couple of months, in Phase 1 and Phase 2 combined, you can hope to lose your first 20 pounds. We will then see this pattern gradually dip, since the body sets up a defense mechanism in the Consolidation phase. However, for the time being, if you follow the instructions to the letter, you should not encounter any obstacles.

Your weight drops in stages

Whereas up until now your weight loss has been spectacular, all of a sudden your scale seems to be stuck. As soon as vegetables are introduced, water artificially flushed out by a protein-only diet comes back into your body, since the alternating phase is by definition less water-repellent than the pure protein phase. Of course, on pure protein days, you'll be delighted to see your scale pointing in the right direction again. You will feel as if your weight is dropping in stages: a little plateau then afterward a sharp drop.

This is the way your body works physiologically. Don't worry. Place your trust in the method. Everything has been planned and organized to make sure you attain your True Weight.

A lot of Dukan dieters tend to overcompensate with dairy products, especially on pure protein days. We recommend you reduce your consumption of dairy products, as these are high in carbohydrates due to their naturally occurring sugars. Dr. Dukan recommends no more than 675 grams or 24 ounces per day.

The rules for Phase 2

Introducing vegetables after the Attack period adds freshness and variety to the initial diet. It makes the diet easier and more comfortable. From now on, a good way to start your meals is with a well-seasoned salad, full of color and flavor, or perhaps a soup on winter evenings. You can then move on to a main dish of meat or fish slowly cooked over flavorful, seasoned vegetables and, to finish it all off, have a dairy product, or two or three!

Alternating pure proteins with proteins + vegetables

During this second phase in your diet, you will alternate periods of pure proteins with periods of proteins + vegetables until you get down to the weight you want.

How you choose to alternate the two depends on your individual situation. Different parameters have to be taken into account, including age, digestion, how many pounds you want to lose, how much exercise you will do, and how much you like meat and vegetables. Rhythms vary from 1 day pure proteins/1 day proteins + vegetables to 5 days pure proteins/5 days proteins + vegetables. We'll look at how you should choose the right one for you.

Whatever alternating rhythm you opt for, you can still eat as much as you want of both the proteins and the vegetables. This "as-much-as-you-want" concept is one of the foundations of my method. The list of foods you are allowed does not change either (see pages 44 and 45).

As much as you want, so you go the distance

Take care that you do not use this argument as some sort of token gesture. Faced with hunger, temptation, cravings, and irresistible urges to snack, having this total freedom makes sense, and it has a powerful role to play. However, it must not be some mere game or a way of keeping yourself busy.

I know some patients who settle down and chomp away without feeling hungry, as if they were chewing gum. Try and avoid this temptation. Vegetables are not that innocuous, so eat them only until you have completely satisfied your hunger. This does not change the principle at the heart of this diet—that quantities are not restricted—and however much you ingest you will continue losing weight, but at a less steady rate, which is of course less encouraging.

Vegetables, yes, but on certain conditions

Provided you choose your vegetables from the list (see page 76), you are allowed all these vegetables, raw or cooked, with no limit on quantity. You can eat them whenever you fancy. However, do take care to follow the instructions about how to prepare them so that you avoid increasing your fat intake, as you must cut out fats as much as possible.

SLIMMING SECRET #5—
EGGPLANT: NATURE'S APPETITE SUPPRESSANT

You're hungry and you like to feel full after a meal. If you are drawn toward foods that are delicious and help you lose weight—then I've got what you need! Take a lovely eggplant and, using a knife, pierce it a few times, about a ½-inch deep on each side. Push a clove of garlic into each slit. Then put the eggplant in the oven at 450°F. When you can hear the skin crackle and you see it's starting to peel away with the crackling, take the eggplant out and put it on a plate. Then cut it in half lengthwise as you would an avocado. Take one half—add sea salt and pepper to taste—then enjoy. Try this before the rest of your meal, it will trigger satiety in the brain. You'll be able to tackle your lunch or dinner more calmly, and the eggplant's pectin will pass through your body taking some calories with it. Life is sweet with eggplants!

Worrying about your weight loss slowing down

Once vegetables are introduced, some patients who up until now have been following their instructions religiously, start to allow themselves an occasional small lapse. Often this is connected with the natural slowing down of the weight-loss process, which had been extremely rapid in the Attack phase.

This slowing down is quite normal and would have come about anyway, even if you had carried on with the Attack phase. There are two reasons for this, and they are related to each other. First, surprised by the intensity of the Attack, the body puts up little resistance to this powerful diet, and it parts with its initial fat reserves easily. This surface fat is unstable and can be lost or regained very quickly. The protein diet is also very water-repellent, which means that as the initial fat gets burned, water is suddenly expelled too. And 1 liter of water weighs a couple of pounds! After the first few days, these two factors that brought about your initial immediate loss taper off. Finally, once vegetables appear, they are a third factor contributing to this slowing down. You are now involved in a quite different and fiercer battle, and you will have to accept that this hand-to-hand combat will take longer.

Bernadette D.—Lost 77 pounds

Don't stop—it's all worth it, and it really works.

"Nothing but vegetables"

As we are following a program in which one of the basic principles is your freedom to choose what you eat and how much, do not fall into the common trap of eating nothing but vegetables. Depriving yourself of proteins would be dangerous. What danger would you run? That of not getting the vital proteins you need, the proteins humans are unable to synthesize and that your body would take from your muscle mass, skin, and hair. When vegetables are allowed, they must not replace meat and fish but should be eaten alongside them. Take a look at the list of vegetables on page 76. As with the Attack phase, take care to stick carefully to your instructions and work on the basis that if a food does not appear on the list, this means it is not allowed.

Alternating proteins
and vegetables

Why alternating is necessary

The Cruise phase, building on the momentum and speed generated by the pure protein Attack phase, is now responsible for guiding you to your chosen weight. This stage will therefore take up the largest part of the actual weight-loss section of the Dukan Diet.

The rhythmical addition of vegetables slows down the impact of the pure proteins. This is intended! You are not meant to keep up too rapid a rhythm, as this would be counterproductive, and it would force your body to put up fierce resistance. Wise home cooks know that trying to squeeze a lemon in a single go does not work as well as having several goes and letting it rest in between. Protein days amount to an offensive, a surprise attack, and this attacking force has to consolidate its position and gather its strength so it can launch a fresh attack.

What is more, the body needs the freshness of vegetables and salads and their vitamins and fiber so that it can digest its food.

What should you do if you want to stop?

A diet is a slice of life that can be affected by unpredictable factors as we encounter obstacles.

- You may get bored of dieting and lose motivation. We are human and therefore fragile at times.
- You may have to deal with pressure, stress, and choices. We are human; sometimes we are forced into things we do not choose.
- You may travel, or circumstances change from when you started, and you have to stop dieting.

In all such situations, one rule must remain inviolable. Yes, you may stop, but stick to the exit protocol. The very worst way out of your diet would be to beat a chaotic retreat. Such disarray would mean losing the results of your hard work. However much weight you have lost, you must keep it off and protect it—it is yours. Go on to the third phase: the Consolidation phase (see page 102). This is a stage you have to go through between hard dieting and not dieting.

How do you choose how to alternate?

There are two main alternating rhythms and two less common ones for more unusual cases.

5 days pure proteins (PP), then 5 days proteins + vegetables (PV)

This is a strong rhythm, often too strong, and it requires unswerving motivation. As time goes by, going for 5 days without any vegetables may seem too long.

1 day pure proteins (PP), then 1 day proteins + vegetables (PV)

In the past, I used to systematically recommend the 5/5 alternation, but then I realized that the 1/1 rhythm often produced very similar results, but without the frustration of 5 days without vegetables, and it also caused less tension. So this is how I suggest you alternate.

2 days pure proteins (PP), then 5 days proteins + vegetables (PV)

This way of alternating is less common and less intense and so is better suited to people who are vulnerable, fragile, older (over 70) and who, in particular, do not have much weight to lose. It is suitable too for anyone absolutely intent on losing weight slowly. Although such dieters are few and far between, alternating like this suits them well.

2 days pure proteins (PP), followed by a normal diet for 5 days

A variation on the 2/5 rhythm is the 2/0—that is 2 days of pure proteins per week, then 5 normal days without any particular diet, but

---

Eat cold food and you'll lose weight quicker

Did you know that when you eat cold food, your body has to heat it to bring it up to body temperature so that it can be digested and, most important, assimilated? Nothing goes into your blood without being heated beforehand. Heating food uses calories, and these calories are taken from the ones supplied by your food intake—it all adds up!

Eating cold food is not always easy, especially in wintertime. However, you can have cold drinks. Whenever you drink 1½ liters of water from the fridge, its temperature is 39.2°F. When you pass this water in your urine, it is now 95°F, so you have raised the temperature of this water by 55.8°F. You have heated it and burned calories. Not many, of course, but they mount up by the end of the year. So if you enjoy cold water, keep drinking it, and if not, have another try.

avoiding any excesses. This diet and pace best suit women with cellulite, who often have a very slim upper body, chest, bust, and face, but ample hips and, in particular, very fleshy thighs. Especially when combined with a treatment, such as mesotherapy, for specific areas, this diet can produce the best results for targeted areas, while sparing the upper body as much as possible.

In this case, it is best to schedule any treatment sessions for those specific areas on a protein day so that any stubborn fat is tackled, freed from where it is trapped, and burned up.

STAYING ON TRACK

To keep your skin glowing and cellulite-free, use a dry brush and brush your legs, arms, and tummy up toward your heart—this technique helps to increase blood circulation and tighten skin.

What can you eat in Phase 2?

During this Cruise phase, you are allowed 100 foods, without any restriction on quantity, time of day, or combination.

For pure protein days (PP), refer back to the list of foods allowed in Phase 1 on pages 44 and 45.

However, for proteins + vegetables days (PV), here is the list of vegetables you can go ahead and enjoy, cooked or uncooked. Don't forget to combine them with proteins.

Bianca M.—Lost 100 pounds

Never say never until you try it!

Vegetables (choose organic when possible)

Allowed

Artichokes
Asparagus
Bean sprouts
Beets
Broccoli
Brussels sprouts
Cabbage (green, red, white)
Carrots
Cauliflower
Celery/celery root
Cucumbers
Eggplant
Endive
Fennel
Green beans
Hearts of palm
Kale
Lettuce, arugula, radicchio
Mushrooms
Okra
Onions, leeks, shallots
Peppers
Pumpkin
Radishes
Rhubarb
Spaghetti squash
Squash
Spinach
Tomatoes
Turnips
Watercress
Zucchini

Tolerated

Goji berries (1 tablespoon on PP days; 2 tablespoons on PV days)

Not allowed

Avocado
Broad beans
Corn
Dried beans and peas
Lentils
Peas

Tolerated Condiments

Cornstarch (1 tablespoon)
Low-fat cocoa powder (1 tablespoon)
Sesame seeds/poppy seeds/flax seeds/chia seeds (1 tablespoon)
White wine (for cooking, 3 tablespoons)

How should you prepare vegetables?

For anyone who can digest raw vegetables, it is always preferable to eat vegetables when they are completely fresh and uncooked so that you avoid losing any of their vitamins.

Despite appearing harmless, dressings pose one of the major problems for weight loss. Indeed, for many people, the quintessential diet foods are crudités and salads, low in calories and high in fiber and vitamins. This is absolutely correct but fails to take into account the dressing that comes with them, which cancels out all of these wonderful qualities.

For these reasons, throughout the whole weight-loss phase, you must only use the dressings listed below:

Dukan vinaigrette

1 tablespoon Dijon mustard or whole-grain mustard
5 tablespoons balsamic vinegar
1 teaspoon olive oil
1 garlic clove
7 to 8 basil leaves, chopped
Salt and freshly ground black pepper to taste

Take an old mustard jar and fill it with all the ingredients, mixing very thoroughly. If you like garlic, leave a clove to marinate in the bottom of the jar.

Dukan mayonnaise

1 egg yolk
1 tablespoon Dijon mustard
Salt and freshly ground black pepper to taste
3 tablespoons fat-free sour cream or yogurt
1 tablespoon chopped fresh parsley or chives

Put the egg yolk in a mixing bowl and combine with the mustard. Season with salt and pepper, and add the herbs. Gradually mix in the sour cream or yogurt, stirring continuously. Mayonnaise must be kept chilled.

Yogurt or sour cream dressing

You can make up a natural, tasty dressing using a fat-free dairy product.

You can even use some ordinary natural yogurt. It is hardly any more caloric than fat-free yogurt, but it is creamier. Add 1 level tablespoon of mustard (Dijon if possible), and beat the mixture so it thickens like mayonnaise and has a nice consistency. Then add a dash of vinegar, salt and freshly ground black pepper to taste, and some chopped fresh herbs.

Ways of cooking vegetables

Steaming

The vegetables you are allowed may be cooked in water or, even better, steamed to retain the maximum amount of vitamins.

In the oven

You may also bake vegetables in the oven in the juices from your meat or fish. Examples of typical dishes are sea bass with fennel, tilapia with tomatoes, and cabbage stuffed with ground beef.

In aluminum foil

Cooking vegetables in aluminum foil combines all the advantages of taste and nutritional value. This is a particularly good way of cooking fish. Salmon, for example, remains moist when cooked on a bed of leeks or chopped eggplant.

"Plancha" grilling

Use a real plancha (flat stovetop) grill pan or a heavy-based nonstick frying pan or a ridged grill pan. This is a fantastic way to cook vegetables as it gives them a different taste and texture. I would particularly recommend it to anyone not overly fond of vegetables. Try it with your children if they turn their noses up at these essential foods.

Brenda R.—Lost 25 pounds

If I can stick with this diet anyone can! The biggest challenge I faced is that I don't cook . . . at all! But I was able to follow the diet without trouble and was never hungry (well . . . except for days two and three when I would have killed someone for a bagel! LOL).

Nowadays, we know that certain spices provide intense flavors, especially cloves, ginger, star anise, and cardamom. They bring together strong, penetrating sensations that work on the hypothalamus, the area in our brain that measures these sensations, until it reaches such a point that the feeling of satiety is triggered. So it is very important to use the whole range of these spices as much as possible, preferably at the start of a meal. If you are not already a die-hard fan, do try and get used to them.

Prescribed physical exercise

Up until recently, I used to strongly recommend exercise, but I did not include it categorically as an integral part of my program. Nowadays, I do not think twice before writing it as a prescription for my patients. Prescribed exercise (PE) is the second driving force behind my method.

Walking as weight-loss medicine

For the past couple of years I have stopped just advising my patients to walk—I now prescribe it like a medicine.

Attack phase	20 minutes/day
Cruise phase	30 minutes/day
Consolidation phase	30 minutes/day
Stabilization phase	20 minutes/day
To break through a stagnation plateau	1 hour/day for 3 days

When you consider all the effort, expenditure, restrictions, and motivation you need to lose weight, what is a 20-minute walk in the big scheme of things? So I am counting on you.

Esteban P.—Lost 111 pounds

We're all human; we all fall from time to time. Don't let it get you down. When you have a cheat or blow it with a big "illegal" meal, just get up and get right back on the diet. Whatever damage was done will disappear again. When you hit a plateau, take heart! Your body is being changed for the better, but it likes to stay in the comfort zone it's always known. You are the master, keep on striving for the ultimate success you seek!

Walking is the activity that:

- is most natural for humans. If we are no longer apes, it is because we stood up and walked;
- is by far the most effective. Walking at a brisk pace burns off more energy than playing tennis, because on a court you only play physically for 20 out of 60 minutes;

- is the least costly;
- can be undertaken at any time of the day or night;
- least injures or damages our joints;
- makes us sweat the least;
- allows us to do other things at the same time—for example, make phone calls, listen to music, even read a book;
- makes us the least hungry;
- can even be undertaken by the obese without any risk;
- you are most likely to stick with for a long time once you have felt and understood its extraordinary benefits.

There are, of course, many other ways of being active—going to the gym, exercise bikes, fitness coaches, martial arts, swimming, dancing, tennis, and so on. However, all these forms of exercise, however useful they may be, are add-ons to being physically active. Although useful, they cannot lay claim to what walking alone is entitled to assert: its universal status as being what all human bodies are built to do. And, as such, it offers the best way of giving your diet a powerful boost.

By walking, you are doing nothing less than adding a second general to your army to help fight your weight problems!

Brianna—Lost 113 pounds

Minimize temptations. Cut them out entirely if possible. Being around things you associate with comfort foods are going to incite a reaction in your body that makes you lust for them. So avoid them, and focus on the fact that every time you turn down an invitation in that first critical month or so, you are ensuring that at a later date, you will be able to go out with your friends. Except then, all the focus will be on how they can't believe how amazing you look!

Purposeful activity as part of your daily life

Purposeful activity involves doing everything you would have had to do before developments in technology freed you from doing them. If you have a weight problem, you need to try and change your attitude toward physical effort. You are not leading the life for which you were naturally intended, and this is making you put on weight. Nowadays, our bodies suffer because they no longer carry out the minimum physical activity required to maintain their muscle function. Not making enough use of our bodies prevents us from burning up surplus calories from our food and leaves us with restriction and dieting as the only ways of avoiding or limiting weight gain. But, more serious, no longer being physically active—what we deem to be progress—deprives us of a part of ourselves, what the Greeks termed our "physical humanity." Our psyche, our feelings and emotions, our physiological equilibrium, and our hormonal and immune systems all feel the effects of this. What we are missing out on will express itself in subconscious suffering that sooner or later will seek comfort in food.

Apart from walking, which is the basis of our natural physical activity, I favor purposeful activity in our daily lives. This is activity that you must try, in part, to wrest back from the machines and gadgets that stop you from being active.

What started me thinking about PE

Two events set the idea in motion:

The first was when standing in line in a Spanish travel agency, I noticed that the three members of staff were seated on chairs with casters. Two of them used the chairs to propel themselves 2 or 3 yards to fetch files or print out tickets, but the third employee always got up and walked. By coincidence, he was slim, and the other two were far from it.

The second was when I was treating a patient who has since become my friend. When I first met him, he weighed over 500 pounds. Once he got down to just over 300 pounds, he decided to give up smoking and stopped losing weight. I was all for helping him stabilize his weight, but he was desperate to lose a bit more. So I wrote him a prescription for a daily 45-minute walk that he absolutely had to stick to. He did it, despite being reluctant and a very senior managing director. Today he weighs about 225 pounds.

Forget about elevators
and escalators (below the sixth floor)

A woman age 30 to 40 who complains about having to walk up four flights of stairs to my office because the elevator is not working is a woman who has "lost her body."

Going up and down 5 steps uses up 1 calorie. Four flights, twice a day over a year, adds up to 1,400 calories, which means your scale will register a loss of over 4 pounds of fat.

Don't forget ordinary household tasks

- Do the vacuuming without sparing any effort. Work the vacuum as you would work the machines you pay for in a gym.
- Walk to the shops to do your shopping, and take pride in doing this.
- Walk your dog.
- Make your bed, but make it properly. Do not bend your back and put pressure on your spine; bend your knees instead.
- Do not shy away from carrying any sort of object or package.
- Whenever you pick something up off the ground, always bend your knees and never your back!
- Do the gardening! This is a great way of burning up calories.

And if you have to choose a few exercises, here are my five favorite ones.

For these five exercises, the watchwords are: build up your muscles, tighten your skin from within, and wait for it to fully retract. Apart from the need to develop your muscles, bear in mind that skin that has become slack after weight loss will need six months to completely finish retracting.

The Dukan special exercises

1. The A-B-C

This exercise works the thighs, shoulders, and back, and you do it in bed, once when you wake up and again before you go to sleep.

Place a pillow at the head of your bed against the wall and a cushion on the pillow to make an inclined plane of 45 degrees.

Settle in a sitting position so that your chest follows the same incline as your cushion. Bend your knees to almost 90 degrees.

Then from your inclined position, sit up straight and then lower yourself down again until you touch the cushion. Try doing this between 10 and 30 times in straight succession.

As soon as you feel your stomach muscles getting tired, change the exercise. Raise your chest using only your arms; this allows you to rest your stomach while your arms continue to do the work. You can keep on doing this simple, quick exercise without getting too tired. Once your biceps start to warm up, go back to exercising your stomach muscles.

Roll on wintertime!

By walking at a temperature of around 32°F, you use up 25 percent more calories. Go out wearing enough, but not too much. Wrap up just enough so you don't feel cold, and you avoid catching a cold.

Start by doing this exercise 15 times in the morning, then 15 times in the evening. Your target is not an easy one to achieve since you are aiming to manage, within a few days or weeks, to do this 200 times in the morning and then 200 times in the evening and in a session lasting only a few minutes.

And why is this exercise so "special"?

It is special because it gets your abdominal muscles moving, and with age they naturally tend to slacken in both men and women. It works the muscles in your arms, where the first signs of flabby skin start to appear. This exercise also gets your thighs, shoulders, and back muscles working, and you can do it in bed. So if you can only manage one exercise, then make it this one.

2. The buttock muscle special

This is another exercise that I do every day immediately after the first one while still in bed, when I wake up and before I go to sleep. It is an immediate, logical continuation and is terribly effective. Having done it for years now, I notice the immediate effects every morning and evening: the buttocks, back of the arms, and thighs warm up very quickly, very powerfully, and I feel them getting toned. Moreover, to my mind the exercise is fun; as you will see, it has a "trampoline" element. Finally, like the first exercise not only does this one work your buttock muscles but it also works the ones on the back of your thighs, your hamstrings, as well as the muscles in the back of your arms. So let's get started!

Start by removing the pillow and cushion. You do this exercise lying flat. Lie on your back with your arms outstretched on the bed. Bring your knees up to your thighs to form a right angle.

In this position, pushing down both on your stretched out arms and also on your feet and the muscles in the back of the thighs, make a bridge shape by raising your buttocks toward the ceiling until your chest and legs are aligned on a perfectly sloping straight line. Once you are aligned, lower yourself quickly, bounce off the mattress and go up again until you form a straight line again. The trampoline effect makes the exercise easier and helps you to keep going until you feel warmth and tone creeping into the back of your arms, your thighs, and buttocks. This is a major exercise.

Again, start off doing it 30 times and then another 30 times later when you go to bed. Sixty times a day will not take more than a minute and a half as you do one after the other. If you cannot manage 30 times, this means your pelvis and backside are very heavy and your muscle base in particular is weak or atrophied by a sedentary lifestyle. If this is the case, do not worry. Do a little less knowing that these muscles will quickly adapt and that before long you will manage it. However, try to do a minimum of 10 lifts in the morning and then again 10 lifts in the evening, because your difficulties prove that you really need to do this exercise.

Then as with the previous exercise, try and add another one each day so that eventually you do 100 lifts in the morning and 100 lifts at night. By then your chest and pelvis will look slimmer from the weight loss, and toned and muscular through combining these two exceptional exercises.

Carelys H.—Lost 55 pounds

Do not give up and do not quit before all phases are completed!! I did it and regret it, and now I am giving it a second go!

---

3. The thighs special

This exercise has a double benefit: it uses the most calories of all the exercises because it works the body's biggest muscle, the quadriceps, which as its name suggests is made up of four muscle sheaths. It also tackles one of the areas most affected by cellulite—the thighs—where weight loss and the flabbiness this causes can make the cellulite soft.

The exercise aims to burn calories and at the same time fill the empty space where the fat used to be with firm thigh muscle. Lots of different exercises target the thigh muscles; this one is the simplest and most effective and therefore satisfies my quest for a single exercise.

Stand, if possible, in front of a mirror, placing your feet slightly apart so that you are firm and steady, and support yourself by placing both hands on a table or sink. Slowly crouch down, bending your knees until your buttocks touch your heels. Then straighten up and return to your starting position.

Although difficult, this exercise produces great results. By definition, how well it goes will depend on your weight, where this weight is concentrated, and how fit you are. If you are very stout—over 200 pounds—you will have trouble doing it once. If this is so, try the exercise without bending the entire way. Do what you can and as you progress you can test your weight loss and how it impacts on your physical performance. As the days and weeks go by, and through practice, the time will come when you can complete the exercise. Soon afterward you will do a second and then you will achieve the ideal number for someone who is overweight, a sequence of 15, which means you are not far off your True Weight.

If from the first day you can manage to do this exercise at least once, you will get up to 15 repetitions in 2 weeks by adding another one on each day as long as you feel able and by not allowing yourself to go into reverse, unless it is to let your muscles recover a little by going back to what you did the day before. As soon as you have finished your first sequence of 15, aim for 30 but take your time; another one every week is just fine.

Once you have gotten to 30 repetitions, you will have firm, nicely curved thighs and eight little monster muscles, four per quadriceps, that will spend their time burning calories day and night. I'll take the opportunity here to give you some good news about your muscles. Whenever you exercise, contracting your muscles burns calories there and then. This you know.

But perhaps you are not aware that once you have finished exercising, the muscles continue to burn calories. Although at a lower rate than during exercise, calorie combustion carries on continually day and night for seventy-two hours and then it stops. This is why it is important to keep going and to link the exercises together; ideally you should be active every single day.

4. The special exercise to tighten arms

This is a special exercise to help arms with skin that tends to go flabby. Most women over age 50 complain about having flabby arms and that the skin on the underside of their arms is going slack or drooping. This exercise will not completely solve the flabbiness, but it will help some.

Stand in front of a mirror and hold a bottle full of water in each hand with both arms by your side. Then bend your arms until they touch your shoulders. Then stretch your arms, bringing them back to their original position. Continue the exercise by bringing your arms behind you, outstretched, and going back as far as possible until you reach a horizontal position. Return to your starting position.

This exercise will tone the biceps found on the upper arm as well as the anterior deltoid, which gives the shoulder its curve as seen face on. The second part of the exercise tones the lower arm and the corresponding part of the shoulder as seen from behind.

To tighten arms that have become somewhat flabby, you will need to do 25 repetitions of this exercise morning and evening.

5. The special calf exercise

This is a special exercise to help with water retention, circulation, and cellulite.

Stand in a doorway, stretch your arms out, and hold each side of the door frame and lean forward while bending your arms. In this slightly forward-leaning position, stand up on your tip toes, as far as you can go, and then go back down again until the soles of your feet are quite flat on the ground.

Carol K.—Lost 13 pounds

This to me is the best lifestyle I have been on.

Repeat this exercise 25 times, take a break, then do another series, then a third and a fourth until you manage to do 100 ankle bends extensions.

If possible, do this exercise once a day. If you have very poor circulation, do the exercise wearing support stockings.

What this exercise aims to do is to get the muscles in your calves (the gastrocnemius muscles) to act like a pump and with each bend to send blood up from the lower limbs into your upper body through the veins in your legs.

SLIMMING SECRET #7—
JUST JUMP!

A trampoline in the form of a mini rebounder might be small, but it packs power—and it does require sufficient space above your head so you can jump. It is therefore ideal for those of you who have a small patio area or high ceilings. If you are one of these lucky people, then try out a trampoline. Increased g-force (gravitational load at the bottom of the bounce) creates a better workout for weight loss, strength improvements, and bone mineralization.

What's even better, it's you who decides how much effort to put in. The more you push to extend your thighs, the higher your bounce. The lower you bend your knees as you push off and land, the better use you'll make of the trampoline's elasticity. The trampoline is about having fun and doing something different!

Some Sample Menus for Phase 2 (Cruise)

	Monday PV	Tuesday PP	Wednesday PV
Breakfast	Hot drink Fat-free plain Greek yogurt 1 oat bran galette (page 48)	Hot drink Fat-free milk Porridge (made with 2 tablespoons oat bran)	Hot drink Fat-free cottage cheese 1 oat bran galette
Lunch	Forester's style salad with spinach, mushrooms, and soft-boiled egg Mediterranean clams (page 194) Rhubarb compote (page 219)	Seafood sticks (surimi sticks) Chicken cutlet with herbs de Provence Dukan cheesecake	Grilled vegetables on the plancha or pan-fried with oil wiped off Rabbit (or chicken) with a mustard sauce and braised chicory (see page 195) Rhubarb compote
Snack	Can of salmon	Fat-free cottage cheese with cinnamon	Fat-free plain Greek yogurt
Dinner	Vegetable protein introductory evening Aniseed-flavored veal stew with fennel (page 197) Fat-free yogurt	Shrimp and cherry tomatoes Ground veal with lemon Shirataki noodles with lemony cream cheese sauce	Steamed mussels Steamed haddock with grilled vegetables Fat-free plain Greek yogurt mandarin cream

Here you are alternating 1 PP (pure proteins) day with 1 PV (proteins + vegetables) day + 2 tablespoons of oat bran, every day.

Thursday PP	Friday PV	Saturday PP	Sunday PV
Hot drink Fat-free plain Greek yogurt Cooked ham (without fat or rind)	Hot drink Egg white omelet with finely diced tomato and cucumber Lean cooked turkey slices	Hot drink Fat-free ricotta Low-sodium turkey slices	Hot drink Fat-free plain Greek yogurt 1 slice gingerbread (page 216)
Dukan shrimp mayonnaise Medaillons of sole with salmon (page 191) with shirataki noodles Earl Grey tea cream	Cucumber and radish salad Stir-fried beef with sweet peppers (page 204) Fat-free, sugar-free natural or flavored yogurt	Eggs mimosa Pan-fried scallops with a vanilla foam (page 163) shirataki noodles with ginger soy sauce Coffee and almond mousse	Cooked carrot, garlic, and cumin salad Roast veal with mustard sauce and oven-baked vegetables Dukan Diet yogurt ice cream with homemade rhubarb compote
2 Dukan Diet Coconut Oat Bran Cookies	Low-sodium roast beef slices	Fat-free milk porridge (made with 2 tablespoons oat bran)	1 Dukan Diet Coconut Oat Bran Cookie
Smoked tofu quiche Marinated seitan kebabs Tofu chocolate cream (page 214)	Mixed salad, with a balsamic vinegar dressing Dukan four-season pizza with tuna Ginger panna cotta with rhubarb compote	Ham rolls with fat-free ricotta Roast chicken Grand Marnier Swiss roll (page 218)	Smoked salmon Tarragon sole fillets on a bed of spinach Iced chocolate soufflés (page 213) Fluffy pistachio mousse (page 212)

The On-the-Go Menu that follows calls for Dukan products at times, but they are not the only options available—you may use other brands provided that all the ingredients are Dukan-friendly. Just make sure to look for nitrite-free, sugar-free turkey jerky and low-sodium, sugar-free marinara or tomato sauce. Whenever Dukan Diet bars or cookies are specified, you may substitute with regular oat bran.

Cruise Phase: On-the-Go Menu

	Monday PV	Tuesday PP	Wednesday PV
Breakfast	Coffee or tea ¼ cup Dukan Diet Vanilla Almond Granola 1 container fat-free Greek yogurt	Coffee or tea Low-fat slices roast beef with fat-free cream cheese	Coffee or tea Vegetable frittata
Lunch	Grilled chicken salad with balsamic vinegar	Rolled-up, low-sodium turkey slices with fat-free cream cheese	Grilled shrimp salad with balsamic vinegar
Snack	Dukan Turkey Jerky	Dukan Diet Coconut Almond Oat Bran Bar	Dukan Diet Mocha Oat Bran Bar
Dinner	Grilled wild salmon and asparagus	Ground turkey with Dukan Diet Shirataki Noodles	Grilled pork tenderloin, butternut squash, green beans

*You may add an additional snack between breakfast and lunch if you are hungry.

Thursday PP	Friday PV	Saturday PP	Sunday PV
Coffee or tea ¼ cup Dukan Diet Vanilla Almond Granola 1 container fat-free Greek yogurt	Coffee or tea 2 hard-boiled eggs 1 cup fat-free ricotta cheese	Coffee or tea Low-fat slices of chicken or turkey Scrambled eggs	Coffee or tea ¼ cup Dukan Diet Vanilla-Almond Granola 1 container fat-free Greek yogurt
Can of salmon over Dukan Diet Shirataki Rice, herbs to taste	Grilled tuna salad with 1½ oz. feta cheese and balsamic vinegar	Grilled chicken and 2 hard-boiled eggs	Can of tuna over Dukan Diet Shirataki Noodles, herbs to taste, Dukan Diet Marinara Sauce
Can of tuna, herbs to taste	Dukan Diet Chocolate Oat Bran Bar	2 Dukan Diet Coconut Oat Bran Cookies	Dukan Turkey Jerky
Grilled trout with Dukan Diet Shirataki Rice	Grilled steak and shrimp, side salad	Sashimi platter (3 pieces salmon, 3 pieces yellow-tail, 3 pieces mackerel) Dukan Diet Shirataki Rice	Chicken vegetable stir fry on a bed of Dukan Diet Shirataki Rice

Fitting your diet into your daily life (Phase 2)

When you are with others, the Cruise phase is simpler to manage than the Attack phase since you can eat more foods. But at the same time it is also more complex, as the temptations are greater and it is easier to lose control.

Eating with your family

If you have children, prepare their starchy foods—such as pasta, rice, or potatoes—separately. Steam the vegetables and put some to one side for yourself. You can always pan-fry the rest of the vegetables for those who want to be more indulgent. For anyone who does not have much time, here is a very simple tip to avoid preparing lots of different dishes. Place the steamed vegetables on the table for everyone, along with some extra-virgin olive oil (full of omega-3s), which the others can use for seasoning. Children just love broccoli sprinkled with hazelnut oil or sugar snap peas drizzled with walnut oil. As for you, you have to eat your vegetables without any oil, so make sure you have all your favorite spices out on the table so you can season them to your taste.

Cocktail hour

If you are entertaining guests at home, you now have a wider choice of foods to serve than in Phase 1. Fill up dishes with vegetable crudités and cherry tomatoes so you can nibble away without any qualms. You have a wide choice, including seafood sticks, strips of ham, shrimp, and vegetables. Once again, the danger may lurk in the dressing, especially when you are invited out. The vegetables already have dressing on them? Then leave them well alone. Of course, if there are any dips in separate dishes, you must avoid dipping your vegetables in them. Lastly, if you are invited to a friend's who loves serving fried food and little pastries as appetizers, then remember to fill yourself up beforehand with a boiled egg or a few seafood sticks, and go for the "glass in hand" tactic: fill up a glass with sparkling water and make sure you keep filling it up so you are not served an unwanted glass of champagne! Having your hands full will also keep other guests from passing you the nibbles.

Greg S.—Lost 112 pounds

Keys to my success: When I eat dinner, I take my time cutting the lean meats up in smaller than small bites and enjoy each one of them. I work out 30 minutes to an hour every day with a purpose. Lastly, I managed through any weight plateau using the Attack phase for short periods during the Cruise phase to help keep the momentum going. The thing I like most about Dr. Dukan's approach is your weight loss is only the beginning of the plan, and his road map takes you the rest of the way to lasting weight loss. Other diets I have tried in the past got me most of the way, but I never knew what to do once I lost the weight. It is never too late to get started. I did it at 51.

At the restaurant

From the menu you can choose meat, fish, and vegetables. Always check with the waiter on how the vegetables are cooked. If they have any sauce or dressing, order a green salad instead without any dressing. If you plan ahead, you can take along some Dukan vinaigrette in your bag to season your meal yourself. Otherwise, try mixing your pieces of meat in with your salad so it does not seem too bland.

Place the bread basket (not allowed) out of your reach. If you like mustard, you can put a little on the side of your plate. Its acidity may help take the edge off your appetite if you have to wait a long time to be served.

Questions and answers

In the Cruise phase, are you allowed fat-free yogurt with fruit?

There is no restriction on fat-free plain Greek-style yogurt, and fat-free, sugar-free "flavored" yogurts are also allowed, "as much as you want." As for fat-free yogurt containing fruit bits or purée, the answer is "possibly, but the maximum is two fruit yogurts per day, provided they contain no added sugar and are fat-free." This can be tolerated if your weight is dropping as expected. If you are shedding it slowly, then do not have more than one fruit yogurt per day. If your weight is stagnating, stop eating them altogether.

Is it possible to eat carrots and beets every day?

Carrots and beets are known for being sweet, and indeed they are. Although they do not contain as much sugar as people think, these are sugars that get rapidly absorbed, particularly when cooked.

If you are tempted to overindulge and eat them too frequently, then avoid these two vegetables.

Christina D.—Lost 35 pounds

On previous diets, if I cheated, I would be so hard on myself and just give up, thinking: *I'm just not disciplined enough to do this.* This time, my mantra has been: *It took a long time to put this weight on, it's going to take a long time to get it off.* It is what would get me right back on the diet plan if I had a wavering moment. Be gentle with and love yourself during this journey, always honoring the place where you are.

In the Cruise phase, are you allowed mustard and, if so, how much?

Normal or Dijon mustard, yes, without any restriction. Whole-grain mustard also works well, mixed with balsamic vinaigrette.

On the other hand, avoid mustards, like honey ones that have too much sugar. If you tend to suffer from water retention also go easy on mustard, as it contains salt.

I have reintroduced vegetables, and my weight loss has slowed down. Am I going to put weight back on?

It is quite normal for your weight loss to slow down, but don't worry, you are not going to gain weight. In Phase 1, eating pure proteins enabled you to quickly lose fat and water. This diet is water-repellent, and the proteins flush out water. When you add vegetables, you are also adding water and mineral salts, so the diet becomes much less water-repellent. You will continue to lose weight, but more slowly, as a little of the water you flushed out is being replaced, which tends to camouflage the fat that is lost. When you weigh yourself, it looks as if your weight is stagnating.

However, alternating in the Cruise phase allows the diet to continue being very effective. As soon as you eat pure proteins again, you will see another drop in your weight. If your scale does seem to be stuck it is really important not to get discouraged, as eating anything you are not allowed can upset the system and provide it with valid reasons to stagnate.

Phase 2 summary

You lose weight going from plateau to plateau

During Phase 2, your body will go into cruise speed. You will not lose weight as quickly as in Phase 1, but going from plateau to plateau, you will lose the pounds you want to. During the first two months, you will gradually lose your first 18 to 22 pounds. The plateaus that you will notice have to do with vegetables being included again and the amount of water they provide. Whatever you do, you must not lose heart when your weight loss slows down, as this is to be expected. If you are experiencing menopause or are at the end of your menstrual cycle, or if you have already tried many diets before this one, your body may also be more stubborn. Do not give in—your body is the one that will eventually relent. The best way of forcing your way through is to walk (1 hour per day for 3 days).

STAYING ON TRACK

Never go anywhere without something Dukan Diet–approved that you can snack on.

And should you feel your motivation weaken

After the euphoria of Phase 1, when you lost pounds as never before, you are going to find that Phase 2 is much slower. The danger comes from having this impression. So you will need to tell yourself, and keep on saying to yourself, that by following these instructions to the letter, you will manage to lose weight, keep it off, and keep it stable over the long term.

And time is not your enemy. Remember that once your target weight is attained, your goal is to learn how to maintain it over time.

So that you successfully complete this stage, concentrate on your instructions rather than on your scale. Copy the list of vegetables you are allowed, do your shopping in advance so that you never run out of anything, and make up suitable sauces and dressings so that no crafty calories start sneaking their way back into your menus. Be objective, and note down carefully what you have eaten in the day; your vigilance will pay off. Tell yourself that the longer the list of foods you are allowed, the greater the temptations, so you run a greater risk of your diet ending in failure. You need therefore to be even more vigilant than you were in Phase 1. Most important, try cooking, even if you are not accustomed to it. Cooking will reduce your frustration with dieting and will reinforce good habits as you move into the Stabilization phase.

Aaron C.—Lost 35 pounds

Men: If you have a girlfriend, make sure you talk things out with her first. Somehow our women often end up sacrificing a lot more whenever we go on diets, but their support will really help you through.

You have had some lapses

What's the big deal? You have lost a day: you add a 30-minute walk to your daily routine, or you go onto pure proteins the next day, and everything will go back to normal again. Don't dwell on it, and most important, don't feel guilty.

STAYING ON TRACK

Remember, if you're in a bind, it's always better to do a protein + vegetables day than to have a lapse.

Covy A.—Lost 74 pounds

Believe. Don't listen to the haters or even the nagger in your head. Believe that it will work. Believe in yourself and stick to it . . . and it will.

You have given up . . . all is not lost

Take a deep breath, and with me at your side, get back on track. There is no question of your being left by the wayside. If you have given up, there must have been a good reason for it. Generally, it is some difficulty or major stress, feeling depressed, or losing motivation. All that matters is that you avoid beating a retreat in a chaotic manner, forfeiting all you have achieved and losing the results of your hard work. These results are yours, and you should protect them. To do this, if you really have to stop, then take the proper exit route and go straight into Consolidation, Phase 3, sticking to the rule that it lasts 5 days for every pound lost. Then go into Stabilization. And as soon as you feel your motivation return, you will feel proud of yourself for not falling apart at the seams, be ready to have another go, and keep on going until you reach your set target.

SLIMMING SECRET #8—
COLD WATER

If you put a 2-liter water bottle in the fridge and let it chill over-night this water will be at a temperature of about 39.2 degrees Fahrenheit in most refrigerators. If you drink it cold, your body will have to heat the water before it eliminates it later. This heating alone expends about 60 calories. It's not a large calorie burn in the short-term, but it really adds up over the course of a week, month, and year!

The Cruise phase in a nutshell

On your menu, you can keep the proteins allowed from the Phase 1 list (see pages 44 and 45), still eating as much as you want.

And now you can add to your menu all the vegetables (see page 76).
How about tomatoes, cucumber, radishes, spinach, asparagus, leeks, string beans, cabbage, mushrooms, celery, fennel, lettuce, Swiss chard, eggplant, zucchini, peppers, and even carrots and beets, as long as you don't eat these at every meal.

As with the proteins, you can eat as much as you want of the vegetables.

Take care with salad dressings; more than 1 teaspoon of oil is not allowed.

You must walk 30 minutes per day and do your Dukan special exercises. If your weight stagnates, increase this to a 60-minute walk for 3 days.

Alternating
In the Cruise phase, alternate between periods of proteins and vegetables and periods of proteins without vegetables until you reach your True Weight.

Choose your alternating rhythm and stick to it.
1 day pure proteins/1 day proteins + vegetables, or 5 days/5 days. If you don't have too much weight to lose, you can opt for alternating 2 days/5 days or 2 days of pure proteins and 5 days proteins + vegetables. For a specific cellulite problem, 2 days pure proteins only per week and 5 days without any dieting.

You will eat 2 tablespoons of oat bran every day.

Consolidation

Once you have reached your True Weight, you go into the Consolidation phase, a transition phase you must pass through between dieting and not dieting.

What you are aiming
for in Phase 3

For every pound lost, spend 5 days in Consolidation

You are going to consolidate the weight you have gotten down to by spending 5 days in the Consolidation phase for every pound you've lost. In other words, if you have lost 10 pounds, you have to follow this phase for 50 days; if you have shed 60 pounds, you have to stick with it for 300 days. But don't worry, Consolidation offers a wide variety of foods and allows you the enjoyment of your two celebration meals per week.

The Nutritional Stairway

Learn to eat properly so that you never put on weight again by climbing up the 7 steps that reintroduce foods into your life.

The "Nutritional Stairway" is one of the key concepts in the Dukan Diet. Throughout the Consolidation phase, it is important the person who has just attained their True Weight reintroduces foods while at the same time learns their value and their importance so that their weight is protected in the future. The Nutritional Stairway is made up of 7 steps, starting with the most crucial one for life and ending with the one that concentrates on pleasure. Let's follow the steps together:

1. **The first step: proteins.**
   In the Attack phase everything started with them. They are VITAL.

2. **The second step: vegetables.**
   They are not vital but ESSENTIAL, because they are rich in vitamins, micronutrients, and fiber, and they are very low in calories.

3. **The third step: fruit.**
   Neither vital, nor essential, fruit is IMPORTANT (1 serving during the first half and 2 servings during the second half).

4. **The fourth step: bread,** which is USEFUL, up to 2 slices a day, in the morning will be best to give energy for the rest of the day.

5. **The fifth step: cheese,** provides PLEASURE and NUTRITION.

6. **The sixth step: starches,** PROVIDE ENERGY, up to two 8-oz. servings per week of your choice of pasta, brown rice, couscous, quinoa (1 serving during the first half of the phase and 2 servings in the second half).

7. **The seventh step: 2 celebration meals,** which are about PURE PLEASURE. 1 appetizer + 1 entrée + 1 dessert + 1 glass of wine. You can have 1 celebration meal a week in first half of the phase and then 2 meals in the second half.

Why is there a rebound effect?

Your body reacts to its reserves being plundered by gradually reducing the energy it uses and, in particular, by stepping up as far as possible the amount it can extract and assimilate from anything you eat. You are therefore sitting on top of a volcano and in possession of a body that is eagerly awaiting just the right moment to replenish its lost reserves. A copious meal that would have had little impact before the start of the diet, now, at the end of the diet, will have far-reaching repercussions.

How long does a rebound effect last?

The rebound effect carries on throughout the whole Consolidation phase—that is, 5 days for every pound lost. Instructions about the length of the Consolidation phase that are too vague, and the euphoria felt after victoriously shedding those unwanted pounds, often jeopardize the diet if this instruction about length of time is not adhered to precisely.

These 7 steps provide you with a way of understanding the importance of the many food groups. This stairway will be your reference tool to help you avoid regaining weight.

A crucial transition phase

During your first two phases, Attack and Cruise, you lost weight and your body fought to hold on to its reserves, but it lost the battle.

While this struggle was going on, your body developed a dual reaction that you should know about: profit + economy.

- **Increased profit:** The more weight you lose, the greater the energy your body extracts from every last morsel of food. At the stage you are at now, this is getting near 100 percent.
- **Greater economy:** The more weight you lose, the more your body strives to cut down on energy used for metabolic, hormonal, and digestive functions.

Jason B.—Lost 56 pounds

During Cruise, your weight will fluctuate a bit, but it will always end up going down once you get back into pure protein days. Subscribe to the website to make yourself accountable every day!

The rules for Phase 3

The whole time you are consolidating the weight you have reached, you will follow as closely as possible the following diet.

Debbie B.—Lost 90 pounds

Do not give into temptation! It really isn't worth it. After all, once you hit your True Weight your reward will be waiting for you.

Length: 5 days for every pound lost

Keep in mind that half of all diets fail in the first three months after dieters achieve their target weight.

The Consolidation phase offers you a balanced diet, but it's not a diet for weight loss. Following the instructions for Phase 3 means you are guaranteed to consolidate the weight you have achieved. You must follow all of the rules, especially the rule about time: 5 days for every pound lost, which is about the time your body needs to forget about and come to terms with the weight it used to be. During this period, you are going to slowly retrain your body and appetite and give it back a little freedom, but only a little: you are still on probation!

Reintroducing foods that were not allowed, but in very precise quantities

As well as the protein foods and vegetables from Phase 2, you will at last be allowed bread, fruit, cheese, and some starchy foods. However, take note, you must adhere to the strict order in which they are reintroduced and to a set of instructions that are specific enough to prevent you from losing control in any way.

The Consolidation phase has two parts

In order to reintroduce foods at the proper pace, this phase is divided into two equal parts (for example, for 100 days in Consolidation, 50 days are spent in the first part and then 50 days are spent in the second part).

In the first part, you can eat: 1 portion of fruit per day, 1 starchy food per week, and 1 celebration meal per week. In the second part, you can eat: 2 fruit portions per day, 2 starchy foods per week, and 2 celebration meals per week.

1 serving of fruit per day in the first part of Consolidation, then 2 servings in the second part

In practice, this means all fruits, except grapes, bananas, cherries, and dried fruit. Fruit is a healthy food, packed with vitamins, but it is rich, essentially in sugars that tend to be rapid-assimilation sugars. So the fruit you eat has to be supervised, and for the time being, you must keep to 1 serving per day. Think of it as 1 serving = 1 unit, that is 1 apple. As for small fruits, use a small dish so 1 unit = 1 dish of strawberries. For larger fruits, such as melon, cut them in half.

2 slices of 100% whole-grain bread per day

You can eat them at any time of the day: for breakfast, as a lunchtime sandwich with cold meat or ham, or even in the evening with 1 portion of cheese. One portion is equivalent to 2 ounces.

1½ oz. aged cheese per day

You are allowed to eat all hard-rind cheeses, such as Cheddar and Gouda. For now, avoid soft-rind cheeses, such as Camembert, blue cheeses, and goat cheeses. One serving equals 1½ ounces.

1 portion of starchy foods per week during the first part of Consolidation, then 2 portions in the second part

Pasta

The starchy food best suited for our particular use is pasta, as it is made from hard wheat, whose vegetable texture is very resistant. This resistance slows down digestion. Nowadays, you can also buy whole-grain pasta. It is easy to introduce pasta into your menus. However, be careful what you have with it: butter, oil, cream, and cheese will double the calories in your bowl of pasta. Give yourself a proper serving (8 ounces of cooked pasta), and choose a light accompanying sauce made from fresh tomatoes, onions, and spices.

Couscous, polenta, and bulgur wheat

You are allowed 8-ounce servings. Serve with meat and vegetables.

Brown rice

This is as good to eat as white rice, and you are allowed one 8-ounce serving. However, wait a while longer before eating white rice and potatoes, as they contain sugars that, for the time being, get assimilated a little too "rapidly." Portions must not exceed 4 ounces.

Lentils

With some of the "slowest" sugars that exist, lentils are very filling and have an extremely high iron content. You are allowed one 8-ounce serving, but do not add any fat. Kidney beans, dried peas, and split peas are also allowed in the same amounts and without any fat.

1 portion of leg of lamb or baked ham per week

Avoid the outer slice of your leg of lamb, as it is too fatty, and if overcooked, this surface fat

Cooking your couscous without adding fat

Place the couscous in a terracotta dish, mix a stock cube with some water to give it flavor, and pour this over the couscous, covering it and leaving at least 3 inches of water above. Let the couscous soak this up and swell for 20 seconds, then cook it in a microwave oven on high for 1 minute. Remove the dish from the microwave, and fluff the couscous up with a fork to get rid of any lumps. Put the dish back in the microwave for another minute—then it is ready!

Eat slowly and think about what you are eating

Pleasurable foods are included again in this phase of the diet. Enjoy them! Eating them slowly will lessen your appetite, since after 20 minutes, you will start to feel satiated. You can also learn to savor all these textures and flavors that up until now have not been allowed. Get into the habit of taking your time, particularly if before dieting you were used to wolfing down your food.

can be carcinogenic. You can eat cooked ham, but you are still not allowed cured hams, such as prosciutto.

1 celebration meal per week in the first part of Consolidation, then 2 celebration meals in the second part

Once, then twice a week, you will be able to enjoy a meal in which you can eat whatever you like without worrying about whether the foods are allowed. This means 1 and then 2 meals per week, not 2 days per week. My patients often mix this up. One celebration meal means 1 starter of your choice, 1 main course, 1 dessert, and 1 glass of wine. But be careful! You may eat all this, provided you abide by one specific condition: that you never take second helpings of the same dish and that you eat and drink 1 "unit" of everything. Furthermore, celebration meals are never eaten in succession. Leave at least 1 day between the 2 meals to allow your body time to clear out any surplus.

And what about oat bran?

Continue with 2 tablespoons per day.

One day of pure proteins per week

This day of pure proteins will guarantee that you do not put any weight back on. Thus you will only be allowed to eat the Attack phase proteins (see the list on pages 44 and 45), with no limit on quantity and without tolerated foods. This takes a little more effort, and it is the only restriction in this phase. Keep Thursdays as a pure protein day.

Diane B.—Lost 83 pounds

Prepare to succeed, make a plan, and work the plan. Prepare foods ahead so you always have something when hungry.

What can you eat in Phase 3?

At last, the range of foods you are allowed opens up! You are going to enjoy being able to eat certain foods that you have not eaten in a long time.

You are of course allowed the Phase 1 proteins (see the list on pages 44 and 45) as well as all the vegetables reintroduced in Phase 2 (see the list on page 76). In addition, you may eat the following foods, while sticking to the frequency and quantities laid down in the rules. You may eat "not allowed" foods at your celebration meals.

Fruit (1 portion per day, then 2; choose organic when possible)

Allowed
Apple
Apricot
Blackberry
Clementine
Grapefruit
Melon
Nectarine
Orange
Peach
Pear
Plum
Raspberry
Strawberry
Watermelon, etc.

Not allowed
Almonds
Banana
Cashews
Cherries
Dried fruit
Grapes
Hazelnuts
Peanuts
Pistachios
Walnuts

Shirataki noodles and shirataki rice

Bread (2 slices per day)

Allowed
100% whole-grain bread
100% whole wheat bread
Bran bread
Ezekiel-style bread
Rye bread

Not allowed
Baguette
Sandwich bread
White bread

Oat and wheat bran

Allowed
2 tablespoons oat bran per day
1 tablespoon wheat bran per day (optional)

Cheese (1 serving per day)

Allowed
(hard rind)
Cheddar
Edam
Emmental
Gouda
Gruyère
Leicester
Manchego
Parmesan

Not allowed
(soft rind)
Blue cheese
Brie
Camembert
Goat cheese

Starchy foods (once, then twice a week)

Allowed
Brown rice
Bulgur wheat
Couscous
Dried peas

Flageolet beans
Kidney beans
Lentils
Pasta
Polenta
Potatoes (no more than
    4 ounces)
Quinoa
Split peas
White rice (no more than
    4 ounces)

Not allowed
Fries
Potato chips
Sautéed potatoes

Meat (see the list on
pages 44 and 45 to
which you can add)
Allowed
Cooked ham
Leg of lamb

Not allowed
Any fat around the ham
Cured ham
Cuts from along the pork
    spine
Fatty bits from the leg of
    lamb (outer slice)

Hannah—Lost 90 pounds

Please, don't forget the oat bran. It is important! Oh, and
don't be afraid to be proud of yourself. You are working hard,
so it's okay for people to notice. And trust me. . . . They will!

Managing celebration meals

So now you will be able to eat a good meal once and then twice a week with complete freedom. This does not mean "celebration day," but "celebration meal." During these two meals, you may eat any type of food, in particular those you have most missed during the diet's first two phases.

Barbara T.—Lost 41 pounds

Don't be afraid to have a "celebration meal." You are given the tools to get back on track!

Get yourself organized

Your celebration meal can be either of the day's two main meals, but dinner is a better choice, so you have enough time to enjoy it. Plan your week. If you are invited out or if you have friends visiting over the weekend, decide to have your two celebration meals on these two days, when you are relaxing. In the second part of the Consolidation, do not have these two meals too close together.

Two conditions

You are allowed everything, but:
- you must never take second helpings;
- you must never eat two celebration meals in succession.

Get into the routine of fitting a Phase 3 meal in between your two celebration meals. If, for example, you have your first celebration meal at Tuesday lunchtime, then you must not have your second one on Tuesday evening.

You are allowed everything, but only 1 serving:

- 1 starter
- 1 main dish
- 1 dessert or cheese
- 1 glass of wine

Curry? Paella? Chocolate cake? You choose your menu, but just one serving of each course.

Be careful with alcohol; if you have had a glass of champagne while chatting before the meal, then you are not allowed any wine during the meal.

Know how to "shut the door again" after a celebration meal

Contrary to what you might think, the risk from these two moments of pleasure does not lie in what makes up the actual celebration meal, but rather in what you eat at your next meal when you have to be restricted again by certain limitations. The simplest way to tackle this danger is to bear it in mind. Write it down on your calendar for the days following celebration meals so that you program yourself to slip back into the Consolidation phase without any problem.

Give yourself some pleasure!

These unrestricted menus also allow you to learn about pleasure, which you will need to learn how to control again. If before your diet, you had the unfortunate habits of snacking in front of the television or downing whole jars of cracker spreads, these two meals are there to introduce you to a quite different form of pleasure. Savor, chew slowly, take your time, and think about what you are eating.

Two tips to stop yourself from taking seconds

- In a restaurant, your plate is brought to you with all the trimmings, vegetables, etc. You cannot ask for a second helping. Behave at home as if you were in a restaurant. Fill up your plate, but don't take any seconds.
- You can serve everything onto individual plates so that you avoid bringing the whole dish to the table; that way you avoid the temptation of taking seconds.

Pleasure and gluttony are two totally different ways of appreciating food. Here we want to open the door to pleasure, not to taking in food in a chaotic fashion. If you eat compulsively, this is bound to ruin your diet in the long term.

Pure Protein Thursdays

Throughout this day, you will only eat proteins that are as pure as possible, as if you were in Phase 1 of your diet. So the list of foods you are allowed is the Phase 1 list (see pages 44 and 45).

Why choose Thursdays?

I chose Thursdays randomly. If Thursdays simply do not suit you because of the way your work is organized, or if eating pure proteins is likely to prove difficult on that day, you may select a different day, but make sure you decide upon a day once and for all and that you stick to it. If your pure proteins day becomes a moveable feast, then the whole Consolidation phase will be at risk.

Elena R.—Lost 40 pounds

Keep lots of protein snacks around. If you are hungry, reach for protein.

What if I haven't been able to stick to my Protein Thursday?

It may so happen that on one particular week the Protein Thursday diet becomes impossible, but make sure this does not turn into a habit. If you were unable to keep to it, then make up for this the following day. However, be aware that it is only a short step from shifting the day around to giving up altogether. Another solution would be to anticipate any problem. If you can see from your calendar that a Thursday is taken up with a business lunch or dinner with friends, then schedule your protein day for the Wednesday. This way, you are still in control of your diet schedule. But here again, remember that your body loves habit and hates unpredictability. The more regular your eating patterns are throughout your week, the less risk you run with regard to the well-known rebound effect that we talked about on page 100.

Why is this day so crucial?

The Consolidation phase is a tricky one. The rebound effect can occur at any moment until such time as you have gotten through this phase, which will be that much longer if you have lost a lot of weight. This protein day acts like a rampart, protecting you against the rebound effect, and it helps you to stabilize your weight. So it is not under any circumstances negotiable. Do not forget that this Consolidation period is a phase when your body will react in an extreme way. If you make the slightest false move, the rebound effect will come into play. Pure Protein Thursdays keep you safe.

Think fish!

Fish contains fewer calories than meat. In fact, lean fish, such as sole, tilapia, cod, and orange roughy have only 100 calories per 3½ ounces, whereas the leanest beef still provides 160 calories. As for the fattiest fish, such as salmon and mackerel, they do not exceed 200 calories per 3½ ounces, while fatty meat contains around 340 calories, and certain cuts of pork contain as much as 480 calories. The fattiest fish therefore often provides fewer calories than an ordinary beef steak. Because of this, fish is particularly recommended for weight-loss diets, as long as it is never fried, since this sends the calories soaring.

Thursdays, for life

You might as well come to terms with this here and now, as we will see in the Stabilization phase that pure Protein Thursdays are the only non-negotiable instruction that you will have to stick to forever once you have finished this book and ended your diet. You have been overweight and your body remembers this. For the time being, let's say that your body is "on probation." Later on, in the Stabilization phase, you will be free to eat again as you want to, but you should never forget that for a period in your life your body has been different. These Thursdays are going to enable you to live normally, to avoid putting weight back on, and to eat like everyone else. However—and you might as well resign yourself to this now—Thursdays will not disappear from your horizon, because they support and watch over those pounds from your past.

Some Sample Menus for Phase 3 (Consolidation)

1 fruit a day, 1 portion starchy foods, and 1 celebration meal per week (this will double in the second part)

	Monday PV	Tuesday PV	Wednesday PV
Breakfast	Hot drink 2 slices whole-grain bread + 1 tablespoon Dukan Hazelnut Spread Fat-free milk 1½ oz. Cheddar cheese	Hot drink 3 Dukan Diet Coconut Oat Bran Cookies Fat-free cream cheese Low-sodium turkey slices	Hot drink 2 slices whole-grain bread 1 oat bran galette (see page 48) Low-sodium roast beef slices
Lunch	Tzatziki Roast pork tenderloin or leg of lamb with green beans Spaghetti Bolognese 1½ oz. Manchego cheese	Mixed salad with shrimp Grilled steak with oven-baked provençal tomatoes Fat-free cottage cheese with cinnamon	Tofu and oat bran tartlets Tomatoes stuffed with ground beef 1 melon portion
Snack	Cooked, lean chicken slices + Dukan sandwich bread	2 slices whole-grain bread + fat-free cream cheese	1½ oz. Manchego cheese
Dinner	Carrot salad with lemon Eggplant and tofu lasagna (page 203) Vanilla-hazelnut crème brûlée with strawberries (page 221)	Ratatouille Coconut chicken with green beans and tofu (page 208) Strawberry and vanilla soy pudding (page 227)	Mixed green salad Chicken and shrimp in a spicy coconut sauce (page 209) Chocolate tofu mousse

Don't forget your 2 tablespoons of oat bran, every day (included in these menus)

Thursday PP	Friday PV	Saturday PV	Sunday PV
Hot drink	Hot drink	Hot drink	Hot drink
Fat-free ricotta cheese	2 slices whole-grain bread	Fat-free cottage cheese	2 slices whole-grain bread
Fat-free cottage cheese	2 slices whole-grain bread	Fat-free plain Greek yogurt	
1½ oz. Swiss cheese	1 soft-boiled egg		
Smoked salmon with scrambled eggs (page 160)	Beet and celery salad	Tomato salad	Vegetable selection with apple cider vinegar
Roast chicken drumstick with shirataki noodles cooked with a low-salt stock cube	Ham wrapped chicory with Dukan béchamel sauce	Normandy-style scallops (page 207) and shirataki noodles in a lemon & ginger sauce	Vanilla panna cotta, with raspberries and balsamic syrup (page 226)
Fat-free plain Greek yogurt sweetened with stevia and cinnamon	1½ oz. Edam cheese	Cinnamon baked apple	
Seafood sticks (surimi sticks)	Oat bran galette with low-fat cocoa powder	Porridge (made with 2 tablespoons oat bran)	3 Dukan Diet Coconut Oat Bran Cookies
Broth-based soup	Sliced fennel salad with lemon	CELEBRATION MEAL	Tuna tartare (page 174)
Oven-baked mackerel stuffed with herbs and preserved lemons	Zucchini stuffed with chicken breast meat	Tortilla chips and guacamole	Grilled tuna and grilled Mediterranean vegetables
Fat-free plain yogurt with vanilla extract and stevia	Apricot clafoutis (page 224)	Chicken fajitas	Floating islands with a hint of mocha (page 229)
		Chocolate brownie	1 glass of wine

Consolidation Phase: On-the-Go Menu

The On-the-Go Menu that follows calls for Dukan products at times, but they are not the only options available—you may use other brands provided that all the ingredients are Dukan-friendly. Just make sure to look for nitrite-

	Monday PV	Tuesday PV	Wednesday PV
Breakfast	Coffee or tea ¼ cup Dukan Diet Vanilla-Almond Granola 1 cup fat-free milk	Coffee or tea 2 slices whole grain bread toasted with 1½ oz. cheese 1 cup berries	Coffee or tea 2 hard-boiled eggs 2 slices whole grain toast 1 apple
Lunch	Grilled chicken on whole grain bread, mustard, tomato, and lettuce	Quinoa with roasted vegetables and wild salmon	Grilled shrimp salad with balsamic vinegar and 1½ oz. cheese
Snack	1 pear and 1½ oz. cheese	Dukan Diet Coconut Almond Oat Bran Bar	Dukan Diet Mocha Oat Bran Bar
Dinner	Grilled wild salmon and asparagus	Ground turkey with Dukan Diet Shirataki Noodles, Dukan Diet Marinara Sauce	Grilled pork tenderloin, butternut squash slice, green beans

*You may add an additional snack between breakfast and lunch if you are hungry.

free, sugar-free turkey jerky and low-sodium, sugar-free marinara or tomato sauce. Whenever Dukan Diet bars or cookies are specified, you may substitute with regular oat bran.

Thursday PP	Friday PV	Saturday PV	Sunday PV
Coffee or tea	Coffee or tea	Coffee or tea	Coffee or tea
¼ cup Dukan Diet Vanilla Almond Granola 1 container fat-free Greek yogurt	2 hard-boiled eggs 2 slices whole grain toast	Low-fat slices of chicken or turkey with fat-free cream cheese on 2 slices whole grain bread	¼ cup Dukan Diet Vanilla-Almond Granola 1 container fat-free Greek yogurt
Can of salmon over Dukan Diet Shirataki Rice, herbs to taste	Grilled tuna salad with 1½ oz. feta cheese and balsamic vinegar 1 plum	Grilled chicken salad with 1½ oz. cheese 1 grapefruit	Can of tuna over Dukan Diet Shirataki Noodles, Dukan Diet Marinara Sauce
Dukan Turkey Jerky	Dukan Diet Chocolate Oat Bran Bar	2 Dukan Diet Coconut Oat Bran Cookies	1 apple and 1½ oz. cheese
Sashimi platter (3 pieces tuna, 3 pieces salmon, 3 pieces scallops, 3 pieces yellowtail) Dukan Diet Shirataki Rice	Grilled steak and shrimp, side salad	Celebration Meal 1 glass wine Guacamole and tortilla chips Steak fajitas Chocolate cake	Chicken vegetable stir fry on a bed of Dukan Diet Shirataki Rice

Fitting your diet into your daily life (Phase 3)

Eating with your family

At last you are allowed to eat pasta, bread, and fruit, so it is easier for you to join in with family meals. As long as you stick to the quantities, you can eat like everyone else, or just about. Serve the pasta onto your plate before the others so you make sure you do not exceed the quantities allowed. Of course, you will not take any second helpings. If your children are fed up with tomato sauce on their pasta, it is easy enough to provide two separate sauces, and everyone can just help themselves. Go ahead and put some olive oil or fresh butter out on the table; this way you will get your children used to new tastes that are excellent for their health. As for you, have your spices ready!

Jacqueline B.—Lost 30 pounds

Include salad greens and make your own dressing (nonfat as much as possible).

Cocktail time

It is true that you are allowed one portion of cheese a day, two slices of bread, and two servings of starchy foods a week in the Consolidation phase. But when you are having an apéritif, keeping a tally of everything you eat becomes impossible. How many cheese cubes can you eat? How many canapés are equivalent to a slice of bread? It is not worth trying to work it all out. Keep these "extras" you are allowed (bread, starchy foods, etc.) for calm and regular times. You can decide, for example, that you will let yourself have your bread in the morning for breakfast or at lunch with a soup. For apéritifs, as with the restaurant, put yourself back into Phase 2—that is, proteins + vegetables. That way, you won't run the risk of making mistakes. You can have cherry tomatoes, seafood sticks (surimi), crunchy vegetable pieces, sparkling water, and diet soda.

Remember that while you are laughing and chatting with friends over an apéritif, you are not able to keep track of what you are eating. Getting embroiled in some complex calculation is dangerous, as you are likely to spoil your evening and jeopardize your diet.

At the restaurant

So that you don't get misled, when you are in a restaurant, think back to the proteins + vegetables phase, as it is really difficult to stick to your instructions and take the new foods you are allowed into consideration while you are chatting away to friends. Do not allow yourself to be served any bread or pasta. It will be white bread, and as for the pasta, it will not come with a sauce you want. If you think "proteins + vegetables" when you choose from the menu, you won't have any problem. Smoked salmon, for example, is an all-purpose dish you can order almost anywhere. As for an accompaniment, you can always opt for string beans and spinach or a salad.

Wine, bread, and dessert are not allowed, unless you have decided to make this trip to the restaurant a celebration meal. If it is a celebration, order one glass of wine. In a restaurant, you cannot have seconds, which is an advantage since this is one of your instructions for the celebration meals. As for the other days, you have to learn to say no to yourself and order a coffee instead of dessert. Don't forget that you are allowed diet soda—it will help you do without sugary flavors.

For a happy diet, follow François Mauriac's example

The French writer François Mauriac, frail and anything but athletic, adopted the habit of jumping up and down in front of a full-length mirror. He started off with small, gentle bends to get his legs warmed up, then gradually he jumped higher and higher.

I thought this was a fantastic idea, so I tried it out myself. I started jumping, as he suggested, when I felt joy, and I noticed that this exercise made my joy more intense!

I eventually realized that joy, which by definition is ephemeral, lasted longer with this physical exertion. So I then tested out jumping like this in isolation without connecting it with joy. And I became aware that jumping gave me joy.

Since then, I have been finding little moments of joy for myself, and I keep the connection going in both directions.

And at the same time, I am developing my quadriceps, the muscles that use up the most calories, and I am controlling my weight.

Questions and answers

Why do I have to count 5 days for every pound lost?

Why 5 days and not 4 or 3? When I devised my first Attack diet, I achieved results that were spectacular, but short-lived. The pounds people lost tended to go back on again. So I introduced new foods, while continuing to supervise and control. When I checked through all my statistics on weight regain with a statistician, I saw that Consolidation phases were always successful when based on 5 days for every pound lost.

Why reintroduce 100% whole-grain bread rather than white bread?

White bread is not a natural food because of the way it is made, from flour where the wheat has been artificially separated from its husk, the bran. It is a food that is too easily assimilated and is quickly digested. It does not provide you with all the goodness you get from whole-grain bread.

100% whole-grain or whole wheat bread contains a natural proportion of bran, and the wheat germ is also intact. Bran protects you from bowel cancer, excess cholesterol, diabetes, constipation, and, given what we are interested in here, it also looks after your figure. Once it reaches your small intestine, the bran sticks together, trapping some calories that get eliminated along with the stools without your body absorbing them. Whole-grain bread also takes much longer to digest, in addition to making you feel satiated.

Can I eat low-fat cheeses (between 10% and 20%)?

You can, but most low-fat cheeses are of no interest to the taste buds, and you will be tempted to eat more than you should.

How can I stop smoking and follow the diet at the same time without feeling too much frustration?

Giving up smoking is so important for looking after your health that once you have made up your mind, it is right to give this absolute priority. So if you have to make a choice, you must put giving up smoking before losing weight. If you want to do everything at once, this is possible, but managing both successfully is rare. You must give up smoking completely and separately for 10 days. From day 11 onward, you can then tackle your weight at the same time. To avoid being overwhelmed by the frustrations of doing both, you must make full use of one of the Dukan Diet's main advantages, as it allows you complete freedom of quantities. Whenever you are gasping for a cigarette, you can eat as much as you want from the list of allowed foods.

Are my thyroid problems compatible with your diet?

In the battle to prevent people from becoming overweight, the thyroid and thyroid problems pose quite a problem. First, there are people who, unaware of having a thyroid insufficiency or just a lazy thyroid, gradually gain weight. By the time they have found this out, the extra pounds are well established.

There are also people who have been diagnosed with a thyroid deficiency. They are given levothyroxine replacement therapy, but often this takes a long time to take effect, so the body continues storing away extra pounds.

Some doctors are wary, preferring to take their time with diagnosis and treatment, whereas all this does is allow extra time for weight to accumulate. Even for those people with an insufficiency who are quickly diagnosed and properly treated, it should not be forgotten that what levothyroxine gives them is not identical to what their thyroid produced.

Think of the difference between ready-to-wear and made-to-measure clothing. This is just to make you aware of the complexity of the problem. If people want to lose weight, with the right treatment that fits in with how their thyroid function is progressing, they will lose weight, that I can assure you. However, let's say that people with thyroid problems must be taken a little more seriously than others, just a little more seriously, but no more.

Phase 3 summary

It is most important that you do not neglect this stage

During phases 1 and 2, you found positive encouragement every day, as you could see from your scales that your weight was dropping. In the Consolidation phase, your weight no longer drops, so it is easy to drift and consider skipping this stage. Whatever you do, don't put this book down! You are only halfway there! If you ignore the instructions in this phase, your pounds are bound to pile back on, and very quickly too.

JB L.—Lost 102 pounds

Know that you deserve this and that you can do anything you put your mind to. This lifestyle will truly change your life forever!

Remain vigilant—the success of your diet depends on this Consolidation phase

You may react in another way by following the Consolidation phase, but only halfheartedly: an extra slice of bread here, another piece of fruit there, three celebration meals instead of two, and so on. Remain vigilant and, most important, be totally objective about what you do eat. Some people on the diet are surprised to see their scales go up when they "had been following the instructions." If you are afraid of making this mistake, write down all the foods you are allowed in a little notebook, and also note down everything you have eaten in the day. Be completely honest with yourself. Don't leave out any of your little snacks if you were unable to resist a food you are not allowed.

Tell yourself that this is your last diet

Going on diets one after the other is bad for two reasons:

- First of all, your body gets used to successive diets. It soon notices any attempts to restrict intake, and so it immediately sets about better managing its reserves! A person who sheds weight and then puts it back on again several times in his or her life becomes vaccinated against losing weight. After each time he or she fails, he or she will find it more difficult to lose weight again. Your body keeps a record of previous diets. So if you have kept going right up to the Consolidation phase, stick with the diet until the very end, telling yourself that this is the last diet you will ever embark on.

- But that is not all. Did you know that when you are dieting, the fats you eliminate move around in your body? Once you have lost 10 or 20 pounds, it is a little like having eaten 10 or 20 pounds of butter or lard! A great quantity of cholesterol and triglycerides is moving around in your blood, and these toxic fats can block up the arteries. This is why losing weight, regaining it, then losing it again is a complete disaster for your health. The risk you run from having fats circulating in your blood is of course largely outweighed by the benefits you gain from losing weight. However, be aware of the repercussions this may have on your health if you go through this process more than twice in your life.

Take heart!

The time you spend dieting will go by quickly, whereas a great figure will stay with you for a long time. This summary page devoted to Phase 3 is particularly important, as you must be totally prepared psychologically to start on this part of the diet. Whether you succeed in losing weight depends on this.

The Consolidation phase in a nutshell

5 days for every pound lost:
How long the Consolidation phase lasts depends on how much weight you have lost. This phase is not optional. It is compulsory and non-negotiable.

Keep your base of proteins + vegetables, as much as you want.

And add:
- 1 and then 2 portions of fruit per day (except for bananas, grapes, and cherries);
- 2 slices of 100% whole-grain bread per day;
- 1½ ounces of cheese per day.

Go walking every day for at least 25 minutes and look for any possible opportunity to incorporate exercise into your daily routine.

You can introduce 1 and then 2 portions of starchy foods per week and 2 new meats: leg of lamb and pork roast.

And now the time has come for 1 and then 2 celebration meals per week.

You go back to pure proteins 1 day a week, on Thursdays: a day that protects you.

Remember, every day, to drink lots of water and to eat up to 2 tablespoons of oat bran.

SLIMMING SECRET #9—
STOCK UP ON STOCKINGS

If you have trouble putting on and taking off your rings, your legs are heavy in the evenings, and your face feels puffy in the mornings—then you have water retention! And, water retention will prevent you from losing weight easily. If you have water retention, you aren't eliminating waste properly and it will slow down your weight loss. Try blocking a car's exhaust pipe when its engine is running—very shortly, it will stop. If this is a problem you have, there are a few solutions you can act upon. And drinking more water is not always the answer, as it sometimes means more retention. My secret is quite simple: when you feel swollen, don't hesitate to try some support stockings. Not the old fashioned ones that your grandmother used to wear, but the very latest models—indistinguishable from the most fashionable tights and panty hose. Circulation is improved in legs that are properly supported with firm and elastic support—using them gets the blood circulating back to the heart sooner and to the kidneys so they can do their jobs of filtering. If your circulation is bad, the benefit will be twofold. You'll see the results on your scale and in your legs, which will be the first to slim down. Try it. Then go walking—you'll see!

Permanent Stabilization

The Stabilization phase: a new life protected by three simple, concrete, but non-negotiable measures.

What you are aiming for in Phase 4

Freedom again

First of all, well done! If you are reading these pages, it is because you have successfully gotten through the trickiest phases of our diet. By this point, you have not only gotten rid of your extra pounds, you have also safely navigated the difficult days in Consolidation, a phase when your body was likely to play tricks on you. Today, any danger of the dreaded rebound effect is past. You will be able once again to eat more spontaneously, without any great risk of regaining weight. You have had to follow many instructions, some more restrictive than others. These instructions were there to guide you—a lighthouse in the storm. Now you will be able to sail far away from the shores, but I will leave you three compasses on board: three simple, concrete, easy, but non-negotiable instructions.

But what in practice does "freedom" mean?

First, I ask you to keep very clear in your mind how you progressed up the Nutritional Stairway. Once you reach the sixth step, you have a model that would have delighted any human who had been alive during the 99,950 years our species has been around. But for the last fifty years, "eating what you want" has meant eating any old garbage. With this stairway etched in your memory, you can now eat spontaneously while still sticking to the three rules without which you will find yourself on a slippery slope:

- You will keep to Protein Thursdays.
- You will never again take elevators or escalators below six stories. You will walk up the stairs.
- You will eat 3 tablespoons of oat bran every day.

As for everything else, it is vital that you keep in mind what you have learned along your journey. Phase by phase, you have moved from vital foods to pleasurable foods, and now you know how to correctly prioritize these foods. Maintain this habit.

Have confidence in yourself

The great difference between Stabilization and Consolidation is your independence. Today, you have regained your independence, and you are in control of operations. Do not underestimate yourself. Today, you are capable of going it alone. As your diet progressed, the difficult days included, you and your body learned a great deal—the four phases in this diet have enabled you to develop in-depth knowledge about how to eat. You can now differentiate between what is important and what is superfluous. Starting with the protein diet, you discovered the power of these vital foods. You then continued onward, adding indispensable vegetables to this base, and, last, in the Consolidation phase, you were able to discriminate and complete your menus with important foods (fruit), useful foods (whole-grain bread), then comfort foods (starchy foods), and finally pleasurable foods (cheese and celebration meals) and dangerous foods (nuts, spreads, chips, mayonnaise, etc.). Your body has grown accustomed to eating in a different way. From now on, you can trust it and give it the freedom it deserves, if you stick to your three measures and the points of reference from your Nutritional Stairway. This is the minimum requirement to avoid putting weight back on. And this protection, as essential and as active as it may be, cannot allow you to start eating the foods again that were responsible for your weight gain.

Jean Y.—Lost 60 pounds

Never get hungry. Eat all you want of allowable foods.

The three rules you have to keep to for a very long time

Why not forever?

A Protein Thursday every week

From now on, you are free to eat normally 6 days out of 7, but this final permanent instruction will be all that protects you from your tendency to put weight back on. During this day, you will select the purest possible proteins. You may also use protein powders (but not just any old powder), if this helps you. As with the Consolidation phase, this instruction is of course non-negotiable—you must persevere with the habits you acquired during your diet. Choose your day and stick to it. If you keep on shifting it around, you will forget about this day, and slowly but surely you will put weight back on.

A major contract: giving up elevators and escalators

If you are not sporty, do not take elevators and escalators below six stories and avoid using your car for very short journeys: in other words, get yourself moving! To motivate yourself, you can buy yourself a pedometer to count the number of steps you take each day. You will soon notice that if you lead a sedentary life, the steps will not amount to much. So, without turning into a top-level athlete, get your legs working every day as part of your daily routine.

3 tablespoons of oat bran per day

Oat bran offers you three major benefits:

- it aids digestion and protects your intestines from serious illnesses;
- when part of the bolus, it prevents the small intestine from absorbing all the calories in your food;
- in your stomach, oat bran increases in volume and gives you a pleasant feeling of satiety.

Eating oat bran daily is beneficial for your health and will ensure that your newly rediscovered figure is long-lived.

Do not confuse Stabilization with Consolidation

Perhaps you leafed through the pages of this book a little too quickly, thinking that Stabilization and Consolidation were two similar things. If this is the case, then go back quickly, otherwise your diet will be at risk. In the Stabilization phase, the restrictions are very insignificant, since the dieters who reach this phase have gotten past the well-known rebound effect. In the Consolidation phase, everything is devised so as to remove any risk of your putting weight back on. This is not so in the Stabilization period, as the risk has now been eliminated.

Margo K.—Lost 14 pounds

Vary your menu, and weigh yourself only once a week.

Should I opt for foods with reduced fat and sugar?

Reduced-fat foods

Nowadays, nobody would dispute the value of reduced-fat foods. There is clear evidence that people do not eat more of them to compensate for their low fat content. In practice, the foods that have most gained from a reduction in their fat content are part-skim milk, now used routinely even for children, fat-free ricotta and yogurts, of which natural yogurt, the most widely sold, is a part-skim product anyway. Other reduced-fat foods, such as butter, cheese, sauces, and cooked meat products, are of more value to people on a restricted diet or at risk of cardiovascular disease. Excess fat also seems to be a factor that increases the risk of various cancers, such as breast, colon, prostate, pancreas, and ovarian.

Reduced-sugar foods

The benefit of these is less clear-cut. It seems that the body can partly detect artificial sugars, and to compensate, it eats more, so that a taste for sugar continues to be fueled and even stimulated. However, it has been proven that this compensation is never total, and it gradually diminishes with use, especially among adults.

Nowadays, the foods that are of most benefit to the obese and diabetics are stevia, diet fizzy drinks, and proper sugar-free chewing gum. Apart from these particular examples, whatever the type of food, the reduced sugar content is aimed far more at people who want to avoid putting on weight than at those who are trying to lose weight.

Some reduced-fat foods

FOOD	NORMAL	LOW-FAT
Butter	758	450
Camembert	283	236
Cubes of bacon/pancetta	280	261
Emmental cheese	400	216
Ham	169	110
Margarine	758	450
Mayonnaise	710	396
Vinaigrette	658	323
Yogurt	90	45

(full-fat or 0% fat, 4½ oz. container)

Protein Thursdays

Selecting very pure proteins

Protein Thursdays are a small weekly reminder of the Attack phase, with a few slight differences. You will therefore have to maintain the habits you acquired in Phase 1 when choosing pure proteins. For example, as far as meat goes, you will avoid pork and lamb, since they are far too fatty to be considered as pure proteins. On pages 136 and 137, you have a definitive list of the foods allowed on Protein Thursdays. Indeed, given that this Thursday is all that is left to protect you from any possible weight regain, it is important that you select the purest possible proteins. Oily fish was allowed as part of your Attack diet, but here it will be banned on Thursdays.

A little reminder

Try to avoid mustard now on Thursdays, as it is salty. Instead, season as you want, using vinegar, pepper, and herbs. To make up for this deprivation, muster up all your spices.

Cutting down lactose

Now that your Permanent Stabilization diet occurs just 1 day a week, your proteins have to be very carefully selected, and your lactose intake should be reduced.

When the composition of fat-free yogurt and fat-free ricotta is compared, you will notice that for the same number of calories, fat-free ricotta provides more protein and less lactose than yogurt.

Drink lots

In the Attack phase, we recommended that you drink at least 1½ liters of water a day. For these stabilizing Thursdays, we advise you to increase the dose and drink 2 liters a day, so your body can really clean out its system.

Cut down on salt

The whole time you are losing weight and consolidating, the Dukan Diet only stipulates "cutting down" on salt. For the Stabilization phase Thursdays, this instruction will be stepped up, as now there must be much less salt on this "protection" day.

Being limited to an occasional single day, this restriction is not enough to lower your blood pressure, but it will allow the water that you take in to pass quickly through your body and cleanse it out. This instruction will be of particular benefit to women who are strongly influenced by their hormones, which cause massive water retention throughout their menstrual cycle.

STAYING ON TRACK

When you do salt your food, use a little Celtic or Himalayan sea salt for instant electrolytes.

You are allowed protein powders occasionally

Even though this is an artificial way of eating, protein powders do have the advantage of being particularly pure. In the Stabilization phase, once the diet only takes up 1 day a week, it is possible to make use of them, especially if you are traveling or if a busy workload means you risk missing a Protein Thursday. As they come in powder form, they are definitely easy to carry around with you. However, you must not lose sight of the fact that these are artificial foods. Your body is not naturally programmed to feed itself with powder. Even when it is flavored and sweetened, powder is not a pleasurable food. What's more, as these mixes contain no fiber whatsoever, they may cause unpleasant abdominal bloating. So you must only eat them very occasionally.

If you do buy powder, be careful not to mistake meal replacements for protein powders. Read the labels carefully. Any powder you choose must be made from whey, soy, or brown rice.

STAYING ON TRACK

Learn how to read and compare labels—be picky about quality and ingredients.

What can you eat on Protein Thursdays?

Thursdays must be strictly protein only. Use foods with the purest possible proteins. You cannot go back to the Attack diet list. Certain proteins that were allowed then are now no longer permitted on these Protein Thursdays. Here is the list of pure proteins you are allowed.

Meat (choose grass-fed meat when possible)

Allowed
Beef tenderloin, filet mignon
Buffalo
Cooked ham slices
Extra-lean ham
Extra-lean kosher beef hot dogs
Ground beef (at least 90% lean)
Lean center-cut pork chops
Low-fat bacon
Pork tenderloin, pork loin roast
Rabbit
Veal chops
Veal cutlets
Venison
Not allowed
Lamb
Pork ribs
Rib of beef
Rib-eye steak

Eggs (choose organic or pastured when possible)

Allowed
Chicken eggs

Poultry (choose organic poultry when possible)

Allowed
Chicken breast (without the skin)
Cornish hen (without the skin)
Ostrich steak (without the skin)
Quail (without the skin)
Turkey (without the skin)
Upper part of chicken legs (without the skin)
Wild duck (without the skin)
Not allowed
Chicken wings
Goose

Shellfish

Allowed
Crab
Mussels
Oysters
Scallops
Shrimp

Fish

Allowed
Arctic char
Catfish
Cod
Flounder
Grouper
Haddock
Halibut and smoked halibut
Herring
Mackerel
Mahi-mahi
Monkfish
Orange roughy
Perch
Red snapper
Sardines
Sea bass
Seafood sticks (surimi)
Shark
Sole
Swordfish
Tilapia
Trout
Tuna, fresh or canned in water
Not allowed
Mackerel in sauce
Salmon and smoked salmon
Sardines or tuna in oil

Dairy products
Allowed
Fat-free cottage cheese
Fat-free cream cheese
Fat-free milk
Fat-free plain Greek-style
    yogurt, unsweetened or
    artificially sweetened
Fat-free ricotta
Fat-free sour cream
Not allowed
Cheese
Whole milk dairy products

Vegetarian Proteins
Allowed
Seitan
Soy foods and veggie
    burgers
Tempeh
Tofu
And
Shiritaki noodles

A few tips

• If you like, eat beef on
  Thursdays.

Beef benefits from being
cooked sufficiently. This does
not alter the quality of its
proteins, but it does get rid of
a greater part of the fat.

• Leave the salmon for
  another day!

In the Phase 1 pure protein
diet, all fish are allowed,
from the leanest to the
oiliest. In the Stabilization
phase, their fat content
means that oily fish is no
longer permissible for
Protein Thursdays.

• Think raw fish!

This is an ideal way of
preparing fish such as
monkfish, sea bass, and
pollock. Cut the very fresh
raw fish up into small
cubes or very thin slices
and marinate for a few
minutes in lemon juice,
adding salt, freshly ground
black pepper, and herbes
de Provence, and you will
have created a quick and
delicious meal.

Some Sample Menus for Phase 4 (Stabilization)

	Monday	Tuesday	Wednesday
Breakfast	Hot drink Swedish crispbreads Natural peanut butter Fat-free cottage cheese	Hot drink Scrambled eggs 2 slices whole-grain bread	Hot drink 1 oat bran galette (see page 48) Fat-free yogurt
Lunch	Tomato salad Grilled chicken with bean sprouts Strawberry and vanilla soy pudding (page 227)	Avocado with crab Sea bass fillets with basil on a bed of tomatoes (page 205) Melon	Shrimps Seafood sauerkraut (page 192) Pineapple with iced crème anglaise (page 223)
Snack	Oat bran galette with low-fat cocoa powder 1 apple	Fat-free yogurt	2 slices whole-grain bread + portion of parmesan
Dinner	Cucumber in yogurt dressing Zucchini pasta with ground beef Portion of camembert cheese Lemony mousse (page 222)	Romaine lettuce salad Neapolitan pizza on an oat bran galette base 2 oz. dark chocolate	Leeks in vinaigrette Middle Eastern meatballs and couscous Spicy compote (page 225)

Don't forget your 3 tablespoons of oat bran, every day (included in these menus)

Thursday PP	Friday	Saturday	Sunday
Hot drink	Hot drink	Hot drink	Hot drink
1 oat bran galette	Porridge (made with 3 tablespoons oat bran)	2 slices whole-grain bread	Oatmeal with cinnamon
Low-sodium turkey slices		Natural almond butter	Apple
½ grapefruit	Fat-free milk		
	1 orange	Fat-free yogurt	
Tuna carpaccio	Mixed green salad	Mozzarella and tomato salad	Radishes
Spicy omelet with fresh mint (page 190)	London broil beef with shallots and zucchini gratin	Rack of lamb with green beans	Roast beef, vegetables, and baby potatoes
Fat-free ricotta with lemon extract and stevia	Mixed fruit salad	Muesli ice cream (page 211)	Apricot clafoutis (page 224)
Chilled shrimp	1½ oz. raw almonds	3 Dukan Diet Coconut Oat Bran Biscuits	1½ oz. raw walnuts
Steamed clams	Gazpacho	Warm goat cheese on a bed of arugula lettuce	Vegetable soup
Grilled sea bass with herbs Provençal-style chicken breasts	Chicken kebabs with lime		Yogurt with oat bran
Fat-free cottage cheese	Ratatouille and quinoa	Fresh herb omelet	
Cinnamon apple surprise (page 230)	Dukan tiramisu	Pan-fried zucchini	
		Rhubarb and apple compote	

Stabilization Phase: On-the-Go Menu

The On-the-Go Menu that follows calls for Dukan products at times, but they are not the only options available—you may use other brands provided

	Monday	Tuesday	Wednesday
Breakfast	Coffee or tea Whey protein shake made with frozen fruit	Coffee or tea 3 tbsp. oat bran as hot cereal Scrambled eggs	Coffee or tea Whey protein shake made with frozen fruit
Lunch	Sliced chicken on whole-grain bread, mustard, tomato, and lettuce	2 slices whole-grain bread with 2 tbsp. peanut butter	Can of wild Alaskan salmon on salad with avocado
Snack	3 Dukan Diet Chocolate Chip Oat Bran Cookies	¼ cup raw almonds	Dukan Diet Mocha Oat Bran Bar
Dinner	Grilled chicken salad with avocado	Chicken stir-fry with vegetables and brown rice	Turkey Chili 2 slices whole-grain bread

*You may add an additional snack between breakfast and lunch if you are hungry.

that all the ingredients are Dukan-friendly. Just make sure to look for nitrite-free, sugar-free turkey jerky and low-sodium, sugar-free marinara or tomato sauce. Whenever Dukan Diet bars or cookies are specified, you may substitute with regular oat bran.

Thursday PP	Friday	Saturday	Sunday
Coffee or tea	Coffee or tea	Coffee or tea	Coffee or tea
3 tbsp. oat bran as hot cereal	Whey protein shake made with frozen fruit	Oat bran pancake, 3 chicken sausage links	2 slices whole-grain bread with 2 tbsp. almond butter, ½ cup berries
Hard-boiled eggs, turkey slices			
Grilled shrimp and scallops over Dukan Diet Shirataki Rice, herbs to taste	Grilled Nicoise salad (olives, potatoes, egg)	Mixed green salad with avocado, grilled chicken, and green beans	Can of tuna over Dukan Diet Shirataki Noodles, herbs to taste
Dukan Turkey Jerky	3 Dukan Diet Coconut Oat Bran Cookies	Baby carrots, cucumbers with ¼ cup of hummus	¼ cup raw walnuts
Whole grilled white fish, herbs to taste, cocktail shrimp	Grilled steak, broccoli, and sweet potato	Warm goat cheese on a bed of arugula, quinoa with cubed tofu, baked yams	Grilled sole, steamed asparagus, cauliflower, and carrots
			Edamame

Fitting your Protein Thursdays into your daily life (Phase 4)

What's this? Are you still dieting?

If you did not notice it before, you are bound to be aware now, that as soon as you start dieting, everyone around you is forever encouraging you to break your rules, using the usual excuse, "Go on, treat yourself!" Food has always been a sensitive topic of conversation. What we choose to eat represents at the same time our culture, our convictions, our childhood memories, and so on. If you managed to avoid this sort of remark when you were dieting, you are likely to face a barrage now that you are no longer on a diet. Yet every Thursday, you are going to eat different from everyone else.

Two solutions for dealing with reactions from the people around you:

- You take ownership and silence any remarks. The way you eat is your business and no one else's. It does not bother anyone, and you are not stopping other people from eating.
- You keep quiet about it. You are not going to explain the Dukan method to your boss at work or to the client you have invited to a restaurant for a business lunch.

Here are a few tips . . .

Eating with your family

Have brunch once a week. Your protein day could be the ideal opportunity for instigating a new family ritual and making your breakfast a bit special: eggs and cold meats for you at brunch is perfect! Whereas the others will finish off their breakfast with toast and jam, nobody will notice you dipping cooked chicken tenders into your soft-boiled egg!

At the restaurant

Order seafood
There is something festive about eating seafood, and no one will notice you following your Protein Thursdays instructions. Did you know that crab, shrimp, mussels, oysters, and scallops are even leaner than fish?

Don't eat your plate clean
Order as large a piece as possible of grilled meat and ask to have this served without any vegetables or sauces.

For dessert, order a coffee
If you order a coffee when the others choose a dessert, nobody will have an inkling that you are on a diet. If the conversation keeps going, then order yourself another one.

What happens if you regain weight? The Flexible Response System

Our Flexible Response System is a way of offering protection in Stabilization. We have developed it to help those people who let their weight slip, despite the protective support their Stabilization program offers.

In practice, there are four successive lines of defense that appear one after the other should the previous one fail to bring you under control and back down to your True Weight.

One key condition: weigh yourself every day

Our whole Flexible Response System depends upon you weighing yourself daily. Get rid of the absurd misconception that leads people to think that there is something obsessive about weighing yourself each day. Not only is this wrong but it defies common sense, logic, and, most important, what we have observed. All the people who have stabilized their weight weigh themselves daily. How can you stabilize your weight if you no longer keep an eye on it?

People who stop weighing themselves are sending out a clear signal that they are scared to step on the scale, frightened of the truth, of the facts, and scared to see confirmation of what they can sense or already know. So weigh yourself each morning.

Try and keep a visual record of your weight curve. There is nothing like it for keeping on top of the situation. You have several ways of doing this: an old-fashioned sheet of paper, an Excel spreadsheet on your computer, or, if you are a Coached member, you can find a weight curve in your Slimming Apartment on the Dukan Diet website.

As soon as you see the first signs of weight regain, get straight into our Flexible Response System. If you get past the first barrier, the second one will go up and so on.

Do something quickly, because it's easier to stave off weight regain than it is to lose regained pounds!

Once you put weight back on, the time you take to do something about it is of great significance. Time is against you, both with regard to your metabolism and your behavior patterns. The longer you take to do something about the weight you've regained, the more established it will get and resistant it will become to dieting or exercising you use to tackle it. If after an indulgent meal you decide that while you digest you'll go for a good brisk walk for an hour, you stand a very good chance of preventing the calories you have just ingested from turning into fat. However, if you wait until the following morning to do something, it will already be a little more difficult, but still possible.

A week later, these excess calories will have become reserves and stored in your surface fat but once again you can still confront it effectively. However, a month later, this fat will be lost in among your deeper fat stores and, infinitely more difficult to access. Only a powerful and well-structured diet will be able to achieve results. To give you a practical analogy, compare your overeating to applying paint to a wall. If immediately after you've brushed it on you decide to remove it, you can do this quite easily because the paint is still wet. But as more time goes by, the harder the paint will get, and once it has dried completely you will no longer be able to simply wipe it off. You'll now need a paint scraper and a lot of elbow grease!

So weigh yourself and take action quickly

But that isn't all. In practice, if you have regained some weight, this is because you have lowered your guard, forgotten about or neglected your protective trident: Protein Thursdays, using stairs, and eating oat bran, either one, two, or all three of these measures that keep you firmly secured at your True Weight.

Why, how, and under what circumstances can this happen to you?

This is almost always due to adversity, constant stress, feeling depressed, an emotional or romantic problem, illness, or problems at work. In a nutshell, you feel hurt and need some comfort. So what can you do? There is nothing complicated or enigmatic about what you can do, but you must not put it off.

Put yourself in a position of armed expectation

Think about the weight you've lost, the number of pounds burned up, the journey that has taken you from your weight at the outset to your True Weight. This weight is your point of reference, the north on your compass dial. Since you do not have the body and lifestyle of a robot, you have **a margin for maneuver that we deem to be 3 pounds** that allows your body to breathe, with its varying amounts of water and food, and for the same reasons, it can breathe socially when you get invited out to birthdays, parties, or business meals.

As long as you don't put on more than these 3 pounds you are still on course. However, should you go beyond this limit, you are starting to drift and your scale should be there to tell you so. Don't go by your clothes or your belts; it is all too easy to think that tight jeans have shrunk in the wash or to tighten your belt by pulling your tummy in. Weigh yourself!

First response, if you've put back on more than 3 pounds—you need to do something!

You've definitely given up your Protein Thursdays; go back to them and double them with a second protein day, either on Wednesdays or Fridays, and do this until you have gotten back down to your correct weight. **Go back to taking the stairs and walking, and add an extra 15 minutes to your normal walk**. And if, as is quite likely, you have given up eating your **oat bran**, start taking it again and increase it to **5 tablespoons a day**. Lastly, drink more; drink as much as 2 liters of still water with a very low mineral content.

Jessica W.—Lost 30 pounds

Don't stop walking and keep Protein Thursday!

Second response, if you've put back on a third of the weight you lost—you need to start a battle strategy again.

Go back to the Cruise phase. Then go into Permanent Stabilization but skip the Consolidation diet. Here too, **go back to only using the stairs and add 30 minutes to your usual walk** each day. As for your **oat bran**, increase it to **5 tablespoons a day.**

Third response, if you've put back on half of the pounds you lost—tell yourself that since the weight regain is still recent, you can still hope to get rid of this weight relatively easily.

But time is of the essence so don't let it slip away. Go back to your Cruise diet, alternating pure proteins and proteins + vegetables, closely combine it with your exercise program, and step up your counterattack by **walking for an extra half hour every single day**, which will greatly improve your chances of success. Once you have gotten back down again to your correct weight, unlike the previous scenario, you will have to go back into the Consolidation phase, 5 days for every pound you have just lost.

Fourth response, if you've put back on three-quarters of the weight you lost—you haven't just accidentally veered off route but rather you are back to your old ways.

In this case, you'll have to go right back to the beginning. Go back to two days of Attack pure proteins, or even three or four days if you have rediscovered your zeal, then start alternating pure proteins and vegetables. How successfully you regain control will depend on how quickly you react and how much time has elapsed from putting the weight back until you start dieting again. However, as part of the Flexible Response System, knowing that measures are in place to deal with your situation and that there is an appropriate solution for it, most people who turn to this do so within a reasonable time scale. In such favorable circumstances, the weight regain is still recent and therefore easier to deal with than during the first Attack phase.

What sort of people cannot manage to stabilize their weight completely or over the long term?

Usually such people are vulnerable and have a history of obesity coupled with weight problems running in their family. They have been emotionally vulnerable since childhood, and this expresses itself in that they are very sensitive to or cannot stand stress. Sensitive, emotional or anxious, and sometimes depressed, they have succeeded in losing weight and consolidating their weight and have started their final Permanent Stabilization phase.

When life goes on without any particular problems, most of these people manage to protect their weight. However, if they are faced with some difficult event, a very stressful situation, the breakdown of a relationship, or a problem at work, then the line of defense may be breached and the Stabilization phase's three basic rules can be temporarily or permanently forgotten.

When these causes of failure are analyzed, a common profile can often be detected. These are people who from early childhood have become accustomed to calming themselves by sticking their thumb in their mouths for long periods or by eating to give themselves some comfort. This reflex steers such people toward reassuring, comfort foods as a way of coping with life's unavoidable difficulties.

In such cases, people need to learn how to stop themselves from automatically eating when they are confronted with adversity. Some people manage this on their own and others need to help themselves by doing some psychological work to learn how to manage their emotions.

Attempts must also be made to preserve anything that can shore up your defenses. First and foremost this means Protein Thursdays, one day a week to fight weight regain as well as painless measures such as always using the stairs, walking, and eating oat bran. Not only is eating oat bran painless, but for most people who are used to it, oat bran is a real pleasure that should therefore be used as soon as any warning signs appear.

Finally, in the vast majority of cases, the weight regain is not total. As soon as the emotional troubles disappear and there is some light at the end of the tunnel, weight stops coming back on. Even better, most people, knowing how they managed to lose weight and having remembered all that they learned, decide to start dieting again of their own volition and succeed in getting back to their True Weight.

As a rule, such people are very well aware of their vulnerability and need to do everything possible to stick with the three Stabilization measures, or with two if this isn't possible, or with just one. Or give it all up if their problems are simply too overwhelming, but then return to the Attack phase as soon as the slightest improvement in their situation appears.

SLIMMING SECRET #10—
A FRAGRANCE BOX

For many, the time between 5 p.m. and 7 p.m. is the hunger trap, the part of the day when those hunger pangs nag away at you. I have a solution for you—find a nice air-tight metal, glass, or plastic box. Place inside 6 decent-size cloves, 6 crushed coffee beans, a stick of crushed vanilla, a pinch of cinnamon, and 2 drops of rum extract. Then allow a day for the different ingredients to meld together and produce a lovely fusion. Each time you feel an urge to nibble something, open up your box and smell the fragrance that escapes from it. Inhale several times—get your fill of these smells and let temptation fade away.

Questions and answers

In the mornings, I take the birth control pill along with my oat bran. Should I take them separately?

It all depends on how much oat bran you eat. One or 2 tablespoons of oat bran are not enough to stop your pill from working, even if it is a low-dose pill. If you have 3 tablespoons and your pill is an ultra-low-dose one, then take it in the evening. If it is a normal-dose pill, it does not matter; you can take them together.

What is the best time of day to eat the oat bran?

There are several different options, depending on your lifestyle and your relationship to food.

If you are a morning person who enjoys a hearty breakfast, it is clear you will find the oat bran substantial, soothing, and filling, especially if you make galettes, crêpes, or porridge with it.

If you are a late-afternoon snacker, then the best time for you would be 5 p.m.

If you grab a quick snack for lunch and never have time to make a proper meal, a large galette made from 2 tablespoons of oat bran, fat-free ricotta, and an egg white can be used to make a Dukan sandwich filled with a nice slice of smoked salmon, some lean ham, or lean roast beef.

If you are a person who snacks after dinner and rifles empty cupboards vainly searching for a treat, a sweet galette with some low-fat cocoa powder is the best idea to prevent you from succumbing.

Phase 4 summary

Those who take it slow and steady go a long way

So here you are at the end of this journey to the center of your body. You gave it a hard time, you waged war on it, but now you can set off again, hand in hand. Your body is your friend; learn how to pay it proper attention. According to an old saying, "He who takes it slow and steady goes a long way." And today there are many of us who unfortunately spend far more time worrying about the state of our car and whether it is working properly than we do about our own body. We would not dream of putting ordinary gas in a diesel engine or of not bothering to take our precious car for a service or oil change.

Kim C.—Lost 120 pounds

**Losing weight and loving yourself is a lifelong
journey; the Dukan Diet is your road map.**

Think about yourself

For this diet to be permanently successful, you will need to think about yourself every day. When you were losing weight, you devoted time to your body. You listened to it, you pampered it or treated it harshly, but you paid it attention. You are going to have to continue in this vein. This is why Thursdays are an important day. This day is a rallying point for you and your body, a time to reexamine your relationship.

Become a tortoise at mealtimes

Taking care of your body means giving yourself some pleasure. Eat slowly, savor your food, and don't swallow anything down without having appreciated it fully. Insist on this, as doing things slowly is a way of life that nowadays is dying out. The more rapidly people eat, the more weight they put on.

Don't have seconds

You learned about this in the Consolidation phase for your celebration meals. Take your time, but never take second helpings. One last piece of advice, which goes some way to helping you rediscover pleasure in eating as well as in your figure, is to eat with a knife and fork. Rather peculiar advice? Today, all our snacking and fast food has made us forget what is so obvious. If you take the time to enjoy a meal sitting down with a knife and fork, you are bound to relish what you are eating instead of gulping down whatever is available through the day.

Joanna D.—Lost 46 pounds

Don't give up; don't ever give up. The tools are all here. If you follow them you can NOT fail.

Drink while you are eating

The idea that this is wrong still persists. However, drinking while you eat does your body absolutely no harm whatsoever. Drinking makes you feel satiated, and it also means that the absorption of solid foods gets interrupted, which slows down the meal as it works its way through the gastrointestinal tract. Furthermore, cold water (see sidebar, page 74) lowers the temperature of any food ingested, which gives the body extra work. And the harder it works, the more calories it uses up.

Karen C.—Lost 63 pounds

Follow the book! By the time you get to Stabilization, you have learned a whole new way of life, and you learn how your body will react to different foods. . . . the numbers may fluctuate, but they will always stay within a "norm" for you!

If you start to put a few pounds back on . . .

Do something before too many go back on. As soon as you start regaining any weight, over just 1 week try eating pure proteins for 2 days, and that should be all you need.

Now, I am sure that you are well enough equipped to face up to the challenge that awaits you as you put this book down, which is to live pleasantly, eating once and for all like everyone else 6 days out of 7. The life you used to have when you felt so uncomfortable in your own skin is now behind you.

STAYING ON TRACK

Drink Perrier or Evian—both have higher mineral contents than other bottled waters.

The Stabilization phase in a nutshell

Disregarding your Stabilization instructions is a surefire way of putting back on the weight you have lost.

You will eat normally 6 days out of 7, in the Stabilization phase.

You will try to apply what you have learned during this diet. You will work out when to eat different foods, depending on how important they are: vital (proteins, vegetables), pleasant (carbohydrates), indispensable, useful, comforting, or pleasurable.

Once a week, preferably on Thursdays, go back to pure proteins.

These instructions are non-negotiable.
They will act as your rampart against possibly regaining weight.

On Thursdays, you will drink at least 2 liters of water.

You will eat 3 tablespoons of oat bran every day.

You will avoid taking elevators and escalators below 6 stories.
Every day, your body will have to be active, even if you are not athletic.

Two major advances
that change everything:
personalization and monitoring

Personalization: an approach with a human face

An international study

In 2003, I set up a network group to conduct an international study on the disturbing increase in weight problems and obesity across the world. Colleagues who are nutritionists in America, England, Spain, and Germany were witnessing the spread of this scourge and searching for solutions.

One fact became obvious: up until then, nothing had managed to hold this weight problem epidemic in check. Opposition to it had been further weakened because research was carried out in isolation, and one method, the low-calorie approach, had been chosen with general approval.

Another conclusion from the analysis highlighted that an underlying obstacle was the difficulty of dieting in a world that constantly encourages us to consume. To overcome this obstacle, help and supervision were required. This was based on two obvious elements: (1) a personal relationship with the people who were going to put themselves through the restriction of dieting and (2) daily monitoring to give them support, day after day, pound after pound.

The Internet, a medium for personalization

All the books, methods, and plans put forward to deal with weight problems, whatever their merits, are standardized methods that do not take into account individuals and their personality, their family history, and their eating preferences.

The "mass personalization" project focused on creating a program that would enable us to carry out a personalized study for each overweight individual. From the questions drawn up by a doctor and colleague, we were able to collect 154 answers to build a profile of an individual case.

Based on all the elements taken into consideration, a comprehensive weight-loss program was suggested to fit with the individual's weight personality—a proper road map. This project drew upon the combined talents of 32 doctors and a team of computer engineers and resulted in us creating the first book in the history of publishing to be written for a single reader.

Based on 10,000 cases, the Apage study showed that treating weight problems using a personalized approach adds a new tool to our arsenal as we fight to eradicate these problems. Optimum weight loss matched that achieved using the best methods available, but the results were radically better for stabilizing weight and maintaining it over 24 months.

Brenda B.—Lost 40 pounds

Stay with the program and be creative and adventurous in your meal choices. It is fun and well worth the effort. The Dukan Facebook page is uplifting and helpful.

Daily monitoring: a pain control program

Coaching on the Internet

Further international consensus focuses on how terribly important daily monitoring is, and, as a rule, a qualified nutritionist takes on this role. However, in France, for example, there are only 270 nutritionists to look after 20 million overweight people. So a coaching system needed to be devised that could be used on a large scale. The only medium that could host such a system and facilitate dialogue was the Internet.

Take care! There are many Internet sites that offer coaching. As far as I know, none of them, not even the biggest sites, provide a personalized service (they make no distinction between users) or proper monitoring (their standard instructions do not factor in results).

Instructions in the morning, then report back in the evening

The same medical and clinical teams drew upon the expertise acquired from the previous personalization project to create a unique service based on new and patented technology: the Daily To and Fro E-mail system.

Each morning, an e-mail is sent with instructions adapted to suit each user. There are three sections, covering food (menus), exercise, and motivational support and dialogue.

Each evening is when personalization comes into its own, along with the integrity of the monitoring, as the users report back with a few clicks on their day's weight, their eating lapses, exercise, level of motivation, and the food they have most missed. Lastly, proving that this monitoring is real, the information provided in the report is then taken into consideration to work out the instructions e-mail for the following day.

It is this patient and constant supervision, through a daily to-ing and fro-ing of instructions and reporting back, that enables users to lose weight with the least frustration and the best results, which are then sustainable over the longest time.

Calculate your True Weight at www.dukandiet.com.

Online coaching is also available at www.dukandiet.com.

Susanne M.—Lost 43 pounds

I started by creating a list of the allowed foods that I liked and knew I would eat, and then I found recipes that worked for me. Be creative with your recipes and don't give up when you stall. It is not the end.

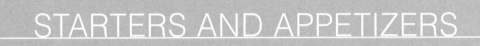

STARTERS AND APPETIZERS

Mini smoked salmon puffs

Makes approximately 50 puffs

Preparation time
25 minutes

Cooking time
20 minutes

For the vol-au-vent pastry
6 tablespoons oat bran
1 teaspoon baking powder
3 tablespoons fat-free plain
   Greek-style yogurt
3 eggs
1 egg white
1 teaspoon bitter almond
   flavoring (optional)

Salt and freshly ground black
   pepper

For the filling
½ cup fat-free ricotta
3 teaspoons fat-free cream
   cheese
Salt and freshly ground black
   pepper
Fresh herbs, such as chives

For the garnish
2 large slices of smoked salmon

Preheat oven to 425°F.

In a bowl, mix together the oat bran, baking powder, yogurt, eggs, egg white, and almond extract. Season with a little salt and pepper and bring the pastry together.

Divide the pastry into about 50 pieces and use them to fill a silicone mini tartlet mold. Bake, in batches if necessary, for 20 minutes. Since cooking times vary from to oven to oven, keep a careful eye on the pastry.

In a bowl, mix together the ricotta and cream cheese. Use a fork to blend it smoothly, then add salt, pepper, and fresh herbs, such as some finely chopped chives, if you have them.

Using a small spoon or piping bag, pipe this mixture into the baked puffs.

Cut the salmon into tiny squares and garnish the puffs. Decorate with more fresh herbs.

Instead of smoked salmon, you could also use lumpfish roe or replace the ricotta filling with a tuna, salmon, or smoked tofu mousse.

In the Attack phase, remember that you should not eat more than 1½ tablespoons of oat bran per day, and during the Cruise phase you should not eat more than 2 tablespoons of oat bran per day.

Smoked salmon with scrambled eggs

4 servings

Preparation time

10 minutes

Cooking time

10 minutes

8 eggs
Salt and freshly ground black
   pepper
¼ cup fat-free milk
3 ozs. smoked salmon, cut into
   thin strips
1 tablespoon fat-free ricotta
4 fresh chives, chopped

In a medium bowl, beat the eggs and season with salt and pepper to taste.

Pour the milk into a medium heavy-bottomed pan and warm over medium heat. Pour in the eggs and cook, stirring continuously with a spatula.

Remove the pan from the heat and stir in the salmon and ricotta.

Decorate the salmon with chives before serving.

Tandoori tofu

2 servings

Preparation time

10 minutes

Refrigeration time

3 to 8 hours

Cooking time

25 minutes

1 tablespoon fresh lemon juice
⅔ cup fat-free plain Greek-style
  yogurt
2 tablespoons tandoori spice
  powder
Salt and freshly ground black
  pepper
1 (12.3-oz.) package firm tofu

Mix together the lemon juice, yogurt, spice powder, and salt and pepper to taste.

Cut the tofu into cubes and add to the yogurt mixture. Stir well so that the cubes are completely covered with the yogurt mixture. Refrigerate for a few hours, or, even better, overnight.

Preheat oven to 475°F.

Place the cubes and yogurt mixture in an ovenproof dish. Bake for 25 minutes, stirring every 10 minutes.

Serve the tofu hot and with cocktail sticks, if desired.

Mediterranean shrimp in a vanilla sauce

4 servings

Preparation time

15 minutes

Cooking time

20 minutes

1 vanilla bean
½ cup fat-free sour cream
2 shallots
2 tablespoons white wine
  (optional and tolerated)
1 lb. shrimp, deveined and
  peeled, tails intact
½ teaspoon turmeric
¼ teaspoon paprika

Split the vanilla bean in half lengthwise and scrape out the seeds. In a saucepan, heat the sour cream until it just starts to boil, then add the vanilla bean and seeds. Remove from heat, and set aside to infuse.

Peel and finely chop the shallots, and cook with 4 tablespoons water over medium heat in a nonstick frying pan until they turn translucent. Pour in the white wine, if using, and reduce a little. Add the shrimp and gently pan-fry until just cooked through, about 3 minutes.

Discard the vanilla bean and pour in the sour cream mixture. Sprinkle in the turmeric and paprika, stirring to combine.

Divide among four small dishes, and serve hot.

Pan-fried scallops with a vanilla foam

4 servings

Preparation time

20 minutes

Cooking time

15 minutes

½ cup low-salt fish stock, or
  water
1 vanilla bean
1 lb. sea scallops
⅓ cup fat-free sour cream
1 generous pinch of unflavored
  gelatin

Pour the stock or water into a saucepan. Split the vanilla bean in half lengthwise and scrape out the seeds into the stock or water. Bring to a boil and leave the pod to infuse for 10 minutes. Strain and keep the pod for garnish if you wish.

In a nonstick frying pan, gently brown the scallops for 2 to 3 minutes. Keep warm.

Deglaze the frying pan using 2 tablespoons water. Stir in the vanilla liquid. Add the sour cream, then the gelatin, stirring continuously, and then strain through a fine-mesh sieve into a bowl.

Whisk the mixture until it becomes frothy.

Arrange the scallops in soup dishes and spoon the vanilla foam alongside.

Smoked salmon parcels filled with shrimp

1 serving

Preparation time

5 minutes

Cooking time

5 minutes

5 shrimp, cooked, peeled, and
    deveined
1 teaspoon fat-free sour cream
1 large slice of smoked salmon
2 tablespoons fat-free ricotta
1 fresh chive

Over low heat, warm through the cooked shrimp for 5 minutes in a nonstick frying pan. Then, at the last moment, add the sour cream.

Place the smoked salmon on a plate and spread the ricotta over it. Arrange the shrimp on top.

Gather the smoked salmon slice into a parcel by tying it up with the chive.

Salmon and cucumber mille-feuilles

6 servings

Cooking time

No cooking required

Preparation time

15 minutes

1 cucumber
6 ozs. smoked salmon
Salt and freshly ground black pepper
3 tablespoons fat-free ricotta
3 sprigs of fresh thyme
1 small jar of salmon roe

Rinse, dry, and peel the cucumber. Cut it into 4-inch-long sections, then cut each piece into thin strips.

Cut the salmon into 24 pieces.

Add a little salt to the cucumber and some black pepper to the smoked salmon. Make the 6 individual mille-feuilles by alternating 2 strips of cucumber with 1 strip of smoked salmon, spreading a little ricotta between them. Pull off some thyme leaves and scatter them on top of each layer. Finish with a slice of cucumber.

Garnish the tops with a sliver of salmon and the salmon roe. Then refrigerate until ready to serve.

Shrimp and cherry tomatoes in a spicy cream

2 servings

Preparation time

   10 minutes

Cooking time

   10 minutes

16 large shrimp
100 ml. (3½ fl. ozs.) fat-free
   sour cream
½ teaspoon curry powder
¼ teaspoon mild chili powder
15 drops of coconut extract
   (optional)
8 cherry tomatoes

Peel and devein the shrimp, leaving the tails intact, and gently fry them in a nonstick frying pan until golden brown.

Make the spicy cream by mixing together the sour cream, curry powder, and chili powder and heating it in a small saucepan over medium heat. Stir in the extract, if using.

Pour the sauce into shallow soup bowls and arrange the shrimp and cherry tomatoes on top of the cream, piercing a few of the tomatoes with toothpicks.

Lobster with eggs and smoked salmon

6 servings

Preparation time

20 minutes

Cooking time

30 minutes

3 whole eggs
1 bunch of white or green
asparagus
½ cooked lobster
3 slices of smoked salmon
½ bunch of fresh parsley,
chopped

Hard-boil the eggs and cut them in half.

Peel the asparagus and snap off the woody bottoms of the spears at their natural breaking point. Cook in salted boiling water for 3 to 5 minutes until the asparagus stalks are tender. Once the asparagus is cooked, drain, place the spears on a clean kitchen towel to soak up all the water, and leave to cool.

Cut up the lobster into medallions and arrange them on a serving dish, placing the eggs on top, with the yolks facing upward.

Cut the salmon slices in half. Arrange the asparagus around the lobster medallions, along with the smoked salmon slices. Sprinkle the chopped parsley over the dish, and serve.

Baked vegetable terrine

8 servings

Prepare the day before

Preparation time

30 minutes

Cooking time

25 minutes

Refrigeration time

24 hours

2 eggplant
5 zucchini
2 red peppers
2 yellow peppers
2 (7-gram) envelopes of
   unflavored gelatin
¾ cup low-salt chicken stock,
   with the fat skimmed off
Salt and freshly ground black
   pepper
1 bunch of fresh basil, leaves
   only
A little Dukan vinaigrette (for
   garnish)

Preheat oven to 350°F.

Thinly slice the eggplant and zucchini.

Place all the vegetables on a baking sheet and bake until the eggplant and zucchini are tender, about 10 minutes. Set aside. Continue baking the peppers until they start to blister and turn black. Take them out of the oven and put them in a bowl with a lid so that they can be peeled easily. Once they have cooled, remove the skins and seeds. Slice the peppers into strips.

In a pan, stir the gelatin into the stock. Slowly bring to a boil, stirring constantly. Add salt and pepper to taste.

In a terrine mold, cover the bottom with zucchini, then arrange the remaining vegetables, alternating the red and yellow peppers, eggplant, and remaining zucchini. Pour a little of the gelatin mixture in between the layers and insert a few basil leaves for extra flavor.

Once all the vegetables have been layered, pour in the remaining liquid and press down the vegetables. Cover with plastic wrap. Place a plate or a piece of cardboard into the mold, put a heavy weight on top, and refrigerate for at least 24 hours.

Just before serving, turn the terrine out of the mold and add a little vinaigrette and a few basil leaves for garnish.

Curried turnip soup with crispy ham

2 servings

Preparation time

20 minutes

Cooking time

45 minutes

⅛ teaspoon vegetable oil
1 onion, roughly chopped
4 garlic cloves, thinly sliced
2¼ lbs. turnips, peeled and
  quartered
1 pinch of curry powder
3 cups low-sodium chicken
  stock
Salt and freshly ground black
  pepper
A few drops of Tabasco sauce
1½ tablespoons fresh lemon
  juice
1 cup fat-free plain Greek-style
  yogurt
2½ ozs. extra-lean thin ham
  slices
2 sprigs of fresh parsley or
  4 fresh chives, finely chopped
1 pinch of nutmeg

Heat a large, heavy-bottomed pot over medium heat. Add the oil and wipe out any excess with a paper towel.

Add the onion and garlic and cook for 5 minutes, stirring often. Add the turnips and cook for another 5 minutes, stirring often. Add the curry powder and stock, bring to a simmer, and cook for 30 minutes.

In a blender, process the turnip mixture until very smooth, about 1 minute. Season with salt and pepper to taste, and add the Tabasco and the lemon juice.

Reheat the soup again, and stir in ¾ cup of the yogurt.

Heat a heavy-bottomed skillet over medium heat, add the ham, and cook until crispy, about 5 minutes. Remove the ham from the pan, drain it on paper towels, and crumble it with your fingers. Serve the soup garnished with the remaining ¼ cup yogurt, crumbled ham, chopped parsley, and nutmeg.

Cucumber appetizers with red roe

4 servings

Preparation time

20 minutes

Cooking time

3 minutes

Refrigeration time

10 minutes

½ large cucumber
6 tablespoons fat-free plain
   Greek-style yogurt
3 tablespoons fat-free ricotta
1 (3½-oz.) jar of red lumpfish
   roe

Peel the cucumber with a vegetable peeler, reserving the peel. Place the peel in boiling water and cook for 3 minutes, until it becomes more flexible. Drain and keep at room temperature.

Cut the cucumber into 4 equal-size pieces and carefully scoop out the seeds so that you leave a hollow about ½ inch deep in each.

Combine the yogurt and ricotta. Fill the cucumber hollows so that there is some mixture piled on top. Top off with some lumpfish roe.

Cut the cucumber peel lengthwise into narrow strips to make ties to garnish each cucumber appetizer.

Refrigerate for 10 minutes, or until ready to serve.

Zucchini pancakes

3 servings

Preparation time

15 minutes

Cooking time

4 to 5 minutes

6 eggs, separated
6 zucchini, very finely chopped
1 garlic clove, chopped
3 sprigs of fresh parsley,
   chopped
Salt and freshly ground black
   pepper
1/8 teaspoon vegetable oil per
   pancake

In a mixing bowl, beat the egg whites until stiff.

In a medium bowl, mix the zucchini with the egg yolks, garlic, and parsley, plus salt and pepper to taste. Gently fold in the egg whites.

Heat a heavy-bottomed or a cast iron skillet over medium heat. Add the oil and wipe out any excess with a paper towel. Drop a third of the batter into the skillet at a time, and cook like pancakes, about 3 minutes on each side. Repeat the oiling procedure for each batch.

Halloween soup

4 to 6 servings

Preparation time

15 minutes

Cooking time

1 hour

1 small pie pumpkin, about 1 lb.
1 medium onion
1 carrot
1 fennel bulb
2 cups fat-free milk
Salt and freshly ground black
   pepper

Cut the pumpkin in half, remove any seeds, and cut the halves in half again. Peel and cut them into small 1-inch cubes.

Peel and finely chop the onion. Peel and thinly slice the carrot. Cut the fennel bulb into long, thin strips.

In a nonstick frying pan, gently cook the onion, carrot, and fennel with 4 tablespoons water. As soon as the water has evaporated, add the pumpkin cubes and enough water to cover. Cook with the lid on for 40 minutes, stirring from time to time to make sure that none of the vegetables stick. If they do, just add a little more water.

Heat the milk in a saucepan.

Blend the soup in a food processor, gradually adding the heated milk. Season to taste with salt and pepper, and divide among warmed soup bowls.

Shepherd's salad

2 servings

Preparation time

15 minutes

Cooking time

No cooking required

4 tomatoes, seeded and diced
2 small cucumbers, peeled and
   diced
2 onions, thinly sliced
2 peppers, stems and seeds
   removed, and chopped
A few fresh mint leaves, finely
   chopped
3 sprigs of fresh flat-leaf parsley,
   finely chopped
Juice of ½ lemon
1 teaspoon olive oil
Salt and freshly ground black
   pepper

In a medium bowl, combine the tomatoes, cucumbers, onions, peppers, mint, and parsley. Season with the lemon juice, oil, and salt and pepper to taste. Serve cold.

Tuna tartare

4 servings

Preparation time

15 minutes, plus 15 minutes
for marinating

Cooking time

No cooking required

2¼ lbs. fresh Ahi tuna steaks
3 tablespoons fresh lime juice
1 garlic clove, crushed
1 tablespoon peeled and grated
fresh ginger
2 tablespoons finely chopped
fresh chives
1 tablespoon fat-free plain Greek-
style yogurt
Salt and freshly ground black
pepper

Cut the tuna up into ½-inch cubes, place in a large bowl, and toss with the lime juice.

In a medium bowl, combine the garlic, ginger, chives, and yogurt. Season with salt and pepper to taste.

Add the dressing to the fish and mix thoroughly. Cover and refrigerate for 15 minutes before serving.

Note: Eating raw fish carries some risk of food-borne illness. Raw fish should not be consumed by the very young, the very old, pregnant women, or anyone with a compromised immune system.

Green chili shrimp

4 servings

Preparation time

10 minutes

Cooking time

3 minutes

4 tomatoes, stems removed
1 fresh green chili, seeds
    removed, chopped
2 tablespoons chopped fresh
    cilantro
Juice of 1 lime
1 garlic clove, crushed
Salt to taste
32 large shrimp, peeled and
    deveined, tails left on

Fill a medium pot with water and bring to a boil. Add the tomatoes and poach for 30 seconds. Remove the tomatoes from the pot, peel, remove the seeds, and dice.

In a medium bowl, mix the tomatoes, chili, cilantro, lime juice, and garlic, plus salt to taste, until thoroughly combined.

Fill the bottom part of a large steamer halfway with water and bring to a simmer. Place the shrimp in the top part of the steamer and cook until they turn pink and opaque, about 3 minutes.

Mix the shrimp with the tomato salad and serve warm or chilled.

Sweet pepper soup with ginger

4 servings

Preparation time
20 minutes

Cooking time
50 minutes

3 red bell peppers
1 red onion
2 garlic cloves
1 (2-inch) piece of fresh ginger, peeled and grated
1 teaspoon ground cumin
1 teaspoon ground coriander
1 tablespoon cornstarch (tolerated)
3 cups low-salt chicken stock, with the fat skimmed off
Salt and freshly ground black pepper
¼ cup fat-free ricotta (for garnish)

Preheat oven to 400°F.

Cut the peppers in half, peel and quarter the onion, and place them on a nonstick baking sheet along with the unpeeled garlic cloves. As soon as the skin on the peppers starts to blister and turn black, take them out and put them in a bowl with a lid so they can be peeled easily. Once they have cooled, remove the skins and seeds. Set aside the onion and garlic.

In a nonstick frying pan, heat 4 tablespoons water and gently cook the ginger, cumin, and coriander for 5 minutes. Add the cornstarch, stirring thoroughly. Pour in the chicken stock, cover, and simmer for 30 minutes.

Peel and crush the garlic cloves. Add the onion and garlic to the soup.

Slice 1 red pepper half into thin strips, and set it aside. Add the other halves to the soup mixture. Simmer the soup for 5 minutes more.

Blend the soup in a food processor until smooth. Pour it into a saucepan and heat it through. Season with salt and pepper to taste.

When ready to serve, add a tablespoon of the ricotta, if desired, and a few strips of pepper to garnish each bowl.

Summer cocktail topped with bresaola

6 servings

Cooking time

No cooking required

Preparation time

20 minutes

3 medium tomatoes
6 carrots
4 celery sticks
Salt and freshly ground black
    pepper
6 pinches of curry powder
A handful of fresh parsley leaves
6 to 12 slices of bresaola*

Poach the tomatoes in boiling water for 30 seconds, then peel and deseed them. Peel, wash, and chop the carrots. Remove any leaves from the celery and slice into small sticks.

Blend all the vegetables together in a food processor and season with salt and pepper to taste.

Pour this mixture into 6 glasses, then sprinkle each portion with a pinch of curry powder and add a few parsley leaves on top. Finally, roll up the bresaola slices and add 1 or 2 slices to each glass.

*If bresaola is not available, you can substitute low-fat or soy bacon.

Pumpkin loaf

8 servings

Preparation time

15 minutes

Cooking time

1 hour 5 minutes

1 pie pumpkin, about 1½ lbs.
3 eggs
10 drops butter-flavor extract
 (optional)
¾ cup fat-free milk
⅓ cup whole wheat flour
⅓ cup oat bran
1 teaspoon baking powder
5½ ozs. cooked chicken,
 chopped into small cubes
3½ ozs. Swiss or other hard
 cheese, grated
A few fresh parsley leaves
A pinch of fresh nutmeg
Salt and freshly ground black
 pepper

Cut the pumpkin in half and remove the seeds. Then cut the pumpkin halves in half again, and peel.

Cut the pumpkin flesh into ½-inch cubes. Cook them in a nonstick frying pan with 4 tablespoons water. Stir occasionally, and add more water whenever necessary.

After about 15 minutes, use the tip of a knife to check whether the pumpkin is cooked. Once the knife goes in easily, remove the pan from the heat. Purée in a blender and then set the pumpkin aside.

Preheat oven to 350°F.

In a bowl, whisk the eggs with the butter flavoring to produce an omelet mixture. Add the pumpkin purée, milk, flour, oat bran, and baking powder. Stir well. Fold in the chicken and cheese. Add some parsley, nutmeg, salt, and pepper.

Pour the mixture into a loaf pan and bake for 50 minutes. The loaf is cooked when a knife inserted into the center comes out clean.

MAIN COURSES

Chinese-style shirataki noodles with shrimp

2 servings

Preparation time

10 minutes

Cooking time

20 minutes

2 garlic cloves, chopped
¼ onion, chopped
1 lb. shrimp, shelled and
   deveined, tails left on
6 fresh shiitake mushrooms
1 cup bean sprouts
2 tablespoons Nuoc mam
   (Vietnamese fish sauce. If not
   available, use an additional
   tablespoon of low-sodium soy
   sauce.)
4 tablespoons low-sodium soy
   sauce
1 teaspoon finely chopped fresh
   ginger
Salt and freshly ground black
   pepper, to taste
1 package shirataki noodles
A few sprigs of fresh cilantro

Heat a nonstick frying pan over high heat and add the garlic, onion, and 3 to 4 tablespoons of water. Lower the heat to medium and cook for 2 minutes.

Add the shrimp, mushrooms, bean sprouts, Nuoc mam, soy sauce, ginger, salt and pepper, and sauté, stirring frequently, for about 5 minutes.

In the meantime, cook the shirataki noodles according to directions given below.

Add the shirataki noodles and the cilantro into the shrimp mixture. Combine all the ingredients thoroughly and cook, stirring constantly, for an additional 3 minutes.

Preparation of Shirataki Noodles
1. Remove the noodles from their packaging, drain thoroughly in a colander, and rinse thoroughly under cold running water.

2. Fill a medium saucepan with water and bring to a boil.

3. Add the noodles, return the water to a boil, and cook for 2 minutes.

4. Drain the noodles, rinse again, and pat dry with a paper towel. Use as desired.

Alternative Microwave Preparation

1. Remove the noodles from their packaging, drain thoroughly in a colander, and rinse thoroughly under cold running water.

2. Place noodles in a microwave-safe dish and cook for 1 minute.

3. Drain the noodles, rinse again, and pat dry with a paper towel. Use as desired.

Shirataki noodles Bolognese

2 servings

Preparation time

10 minutes

Cooking time

1 hour 15 minutes

1 garlic clove, chopped
1 onion, finely diced
1 carrot, finely diced
1 celery stalk, thinly sliced
1 teaspoon chopped fresh
   oregano
1 teaspoon fresh thyme leaves
1 dried bay leaf
Salt and freshly ground black
   pepper, to taste
10½ ozs. lean ground beef
2 large tomatoes, peeled and
   chopped into large pieces
1 cup low-sodium beef or
   vegetable stock
2 packages shirataki noodles

Place a large pan over low heat and add 3 tablespoons water, the garlic, and onion. Cook for 1 minute. Add the carrot, celery, oregano, thyme, bay leaf, salt, and pepper, and cook for 10 minutes more.

Add the ground beef, breaking it into crumbles with a spatula. Then add the tomatoes and stock. Bring to a boil, season again with salt and pepper, adjusting the seasoning if necessary, and simmer for at least 1 hour.

Once the sauce is ready, prepare the shirataki noodles according to directions on pages 172 and 173.

Add the shirataki noodles to the Bolognese sauce, mix thoroughly, and serve hot.

Japanese cucumber and omelet salad with shirataki noodles

1 serving

Preparation time

15 minutes

Cooking time

8 minutes

1 package shirataki noodles
½ cucumber
2 eggs, beaten
1 teaspoon chopped fresh
 cilantro

For the sauce
4 tablespoons rice vinegar
3 tablespoons low-sodium soy
 sauce
1 large pinch of stevia or
 ¼ teaspoon zero-calorie
 sweetener suitable for cooking
 and baking, such as Splenda
2 teaspoons sesame seeds
 (tolerated condiment)

Prepare the shirataki noodles according the directions on pages 180 and 181. If they are very long, cut them up a little.

Slice the cucumber into very thin strips; set aside.

Heat a large nonstick frying pan over medium heat, add the beaten eggs and cook them as a very thin omelet. Remove the omelet from the pan and once it has cooled, cut it into very thin strips.

Prepare the sauce by mixing together the rice vinegar, soy sauce, and stevia (or other zero-calorie sweetener). In a soup bowl, stir together the sauce and the sesame seeds. Add the shirataki noodles to the bowl and let it marinate for a few minutes. Just before serving, add the sliced cucumber. Add the cilantro, and serve.

Japanese sukiyaki fondue

6 servings

Preparation time

15 minutes

Cooking time

At the table, depends on the
number of guests

1 lb. lean beef (preferably sirloin
or rump roast)
1 to 2 packages shirataki
noodles, rinsed and cooked
according to directions on
pages 172 and 173
4 leeks, cleaned and finely
chopped
6 shiitake mushrooms, brushed
clean, tops scored with a
cross-cut
6 spring onions or scallions,
halved, green parts cut into
thin strips
1 Chinese cabbage, quartered
1 (12.3-oz.) package firm tofu,
cut into small cubes
6 eggs

For the dipping/fondue sauce

½ cup low-sodium vegetable
broth
½ cup low-sodium soy sauce
1 cup water
¼ teaspoon stevia or
1 tablespoon zero-calorie
sweetener suitable for cooking
and baking, such as Splenda

For the cooking liquid

2 cups low-sodium vegetable
broth
½ cup low-sodium soy sauce
2 cups water
¼ teaspoon stevia or
1 tablespoon zero-calorie
sweetener suitable for cooking
and baking, such as Splenda

Place the beef in the freezer for 20 minutes to firm it up. Remove the beef from the freezer and immediately cut it into very thin slices using a very sharp chef's knife.

Arrange the beef, vegetables, and tofu on a large serving dish.

Prepare the dipping/fondue sauce by combining all the ingredients in a small saucepan. Bring to a boil, then pour into a fondue pot set over Sterno. Keep hot.

In a bowl, beat the eggs and pour them into a high-sided dish.

In a large pot, combine the cooking liquid ingredients. Bring to a boil. Reduce heat to medium and add the sliced beef, the vegetables, and the shirataki noodles. As soon as the beef is cooked, about 3 minutes, ladle some beef, vegetables, noodles, and broth into serving bowls. Use fondue skewers to dip the beef and vegetables into the dipping sauce and beaten eggs.

6-flavor vegetable and tofu kebabs

4 servings

Preparation time

15 minutes

Cooking time

at the table, depends on the number of guests

1 cup fat-free plain Greek-style yogurt
1 tablespoon fresh mint, chopped
1 teaspoon ground cumin
1 teaspoon ground coriander seeds
½ teaspoon paprika
1 pinch turmeric
1 pinch ground ginger
Salt and freshly ground black pepper, to taste
1 small eggplant, cut into ¾-inch cubes
1 (12.3-oz.) package firm tofu, cut into ¾-inch cubes
1 zucchini, cut into cubes
8 button mushrooms
8 cherry tomatoes

In a bowl, mix together the yogurt, mint, cumin, coriander, paprika, turmeric, and ginger. Season with salt and pepper. Cover with plastic wrap and refrigerate. Place the eggplant and tofu in a colander, sprinkle with salt, and let it disgorge for 15 minutes, and then rinse and drain.

Thread the eggplant, tofu, zucchini, mushrooms, and cherry tomatoes onto kebab skewers.

Place the kebabs in a shallow dish and brush them with the yogurt sauce. Cover the dish with plastic wrap and refrigerate until you are ready to cook the kebabs.

When ready to eat, cook the kebabs on a grill or under the broiler for about 5 minutes on each side. If there is any yogurt sauce left at the bottom of the dish, pour this over the grilled kebabs.

Note: You will need wooden or metal skewers for this recipe. If you are using wooden skewers, soak them in water for at least 30 minutes before using them so they won't burn.

Vegetarian ragout with wheat seitan

4 servings

Preparation time

10 minutes

Cooking time

20 minutes

2 (8-oz.) packages seitan, sliced into small pieces

3 onions

12 whole cloves

6 carrots, peeled and sliced

15 medium button mushrooms, brushed clean and thinly sliced

1 garlic clove, chopped

1 sprig fresh thyme

A few sprigs fresh rosemary

4¼ cups low-sodium vegetable stock

2 tablespoons cornstarch (tolerated)

Salt and freshly ground black pepper

Separate the seitan slices so they do not stick together. Set aside.

Insert 3 or 4 cloves into each onion. Place the onions, carrots, and mushrooms in a heavy-bottomed pot. Add the garlic, thyme, and rosemary. Cover all the ingredients with the stock. Bring the mixture to boil over medium heat. Add the seitan slices. Cover, reduce heat slightly, and simmer for 15 minutes. If necessary, add more stock or water.

Once the vegetables are cooked, ladle some stock in a small bowl and stir in the cornstarch until dissolved. Pour the cornstarch mixture back into the pot to thicken the sauce. Taste and adjust the seasoning if necessary.

Indian-style curried artichokes and mushrooms

4 servings

Preparation time

25 minutes

Cooking time

30 minutes

2 onions, peeled and chopped
1 celery stalk, sliced
1 sprig fresh thyme
1 sprig fresh parsley
1 dried bay leaf
1 tablespoon cornstarch
   (tolerated)
1 teaspoon curry powder
8 ozs. low-sodium vegetable
   stock (or fat-free beef stock)
Salt and freshly ground black
   pepper
12 medium mushrooms,
   brushed clean and thinly sliced
1 garlic clove, chopped
4 artichoke hearts
Juice of 1 lemon
4 tablespoons fat-free plain
   Greek-style yogurt

In a large nonstick frying pan over medium heat, add 3 tablespoons water, the onions and celery, and cook for 5 minutes. Add the thyme, parsley, and bay leaf. Let the water evaporate and vegetables brown slightly. Then stir in the cornstarch and curry powder. Stir well and pour in the stock. Season with salt and pepper, reduce heat to low, and simmer for about 20 minutes.

In another nonstick frying pan, quickly fry the mushrooms and garlic in a few tablespoons of water. Season with salt to taste. Combine the mushrooms with the artichoke hearts and arrange them on a serving platter.

Strain the sauce, then stir in the lemon juice and yogurt. Pour the sauce over the vegetables, and serve immediately.

Shirataki noodles with silken tofu and vegetables

2 servings

Preparation time

10 minutes

Cooking time

20 minutes

2 packages of shirataki noodles
2 scallions
2 garlic cloves, chopped
2 carrots, peeled and julienned
4 mushrooms, brushed clean
  and sliced
1 cup bean sprouts
4 tablespoons low-sodium soy
  sauce
1 teaspoon chopped fresh ginger
¾ cup silken tofu
Salt and freshly ground black
  pepper, to taste
A few sprigs fresh cilantro

Cook the shirataki noodles according to the directions on pages 180 and 181.

Wash and chop the white parts of the scallions. Using scissors, slice the green parts into very thin strips.

In a nonstick skillet over high heat, add the scallion whites, garlic, and 3 to 4 tablespoons of water. Heat until they start to soften, and then reduce heat to medium.

Add the scallion greens, carrots, mushrooms, bean sprouts, soy sauce, ginger, tofu, and salt and pepper. Cook for about 15 minutes, stirring constantly.

Add the shirataki noodles to the vegetable mixture, stirring to combine. Stir in the cilantro.

Heat the mixture for 3 minutes. Taste and adjust the seasoning, if necessary.

Spicy omelet with fresh mint

2 servings

Preparation time

5 minutes

Cooking time

10 minutes

4 eggs
3 tablespoons fat-free ricotta
Salt and freshly ground black
   pepper
1 generous pinch of curry
   powder
A few fresh mint leaves

In a bowl, beat together the eggs and ricotta. Add salt, pepper, and the curry powder.

Chop the mint leaves and add them to the mixture. Stir well.

Pour half the mixture into a nonstick frying pan, cook both sides of the omelet over medium-low heat. Slide it onto a plate to serve.

Repeat with the remaining mixture to make the second omelet.

Medallions of sole with salmon

4 servings

Preparation time

20 minutes

Cooking time

20 minutes

5½ ozs. salmon steak
4 (6-oz.) fillets of sole
Sea salt and freshly ground black
    pepper
Juice of 1 lemon

Preheat oven to 400°F.

Cut the salmon steak into 4 pieces, removing any skin.

Prepare the 4 fillets of sole, removing any bones or skin.

Place a piece of salmon on top of each fillet, and roll the fillet of sole around the salmon. Tie each one together with a piece of food-safe kitchen string.

Place the fish in an ovenproof dish. Sprinkle each portion with sea salt and freshly ground pepper, and squeeze some lemon juice on top.

Bake for 20 minutes.

Seafood sauerkraut

4 servings

Preparation time

30 minutes

Cooking time

1 hour 15 minutes

For the sauce
2 shallots
⅓ cup Riesling (tolerated)
10 drops butter-flavor extract
(optional)
Salt and freshly ground pepper

For the seafood
8 cups sauerkraut, uncooked
10 juniper berries
⅓ cup Riesling (tolerated)
1¼ lbs. cod fillets
12 sea scallops
½ lb. flounder fillets
6 mussels
6 shrimp, shells on
6 thin slices of smoked eel
(optional)
Some fresh dill sprigs (for
garnish)
Freshly ground black pepper
Wooden skewers

To make the sauce, finely chop the shallots and put them in a saucepan with the ⅓ cup Riesling, the butter extract (if using), and 5 tablespoons water. Add salt and pepper to taste. Reduce over high heat until thickened. Keep the sauce warm in a double boiler until ready to serve.

Rinse the sauerkraut several times and put it into a pot with the juniper berries and the ⅓ cup Riesling. Heat thoroughly over medium-low heat.

Cut the cod fillets into 16 cubes and season with pepper. Using wooden skewers, make kebabs by alternating the cod cubes with the scallops.

Scrub the mussels and rinse well, discarding any that are broken or don't close.

Fill the bottom part of a large steamer halfway with water and bring to a simmer. Place the kebabs in the top part of the steamer. Steam for 5 minutes, then add the flounder and mussels. Steam for 3 minutes more, and then add the shrimp and eel (if using). Cook until the shrimp turns pink, about 3 minutes more.

Arrange the sauerkraut on a heated serving dish and place the fish and seafood on top, discarding any mussels that haven't opened. Garnish with the dill sprigs, and serve the sauce on the side.

Cod gratin with chanterelle mushrooms

4 servings

Preparation time

30 minutes

Cooking time

40 minutes

1¼ lbs. cod
1 small bunch of fresh thyme
2 onions, 1 finely chopped
4 whole cloves
2 bay leaves
1 bunch of parsley, chopped
1⅓ cups low-salt chicken stock,
    with the fat skimmed off,
    divided
3 cups chanterelle mushrooms, if
    chanterelles are not available,
    button mushrooms cut in half
    may be substituted
Salt and freshly ground black
    pepper
3 garlic cloves, crushed
⅔ cup fat-free sour cream
½ cup grated Swiss or other
    hard cheese (5% fat)

Preheat oven to 350°F.

Pour 2 inches of water into a saucepan and bring to a simmer. Add the cod, thyme, one of the onions studded with the 4 cloves, bay leaves, and a little parsley. Cook for 10 minutes.

Pour ⅔ cup of the chicken stock into a frying pan. Add the mushrooms, season with salt and pepper, and cook until tender, about 5 minutes.

Add the crushed garlic and chopped parsley to the cooked mushrooms. Stir, turn off the heat, cover the pan with a lid, then leave the mushrooms to soak up the flavors while you cook the other onion.

In a nonstick frying pan, gently cook the other finely chopped onion until softened, then pour in the remaining ⅔ cup stock. Leave to simmer over low heat until all the liquid has evaporated.

Heat the frying pan again with the mushrooms, add the onion and flaked cod, stir, and then stir in the sour cream. Pour the mixture into a casserole dish, sprinkle with the cheese, and bake for 20 minutes.

Mediterranean clams

2 to 4 servings

Preparation time

10 minutes

Cooking time

35 minutes

6 shallots
1 (14.5-oz.) can of diced
   tomatoes, about 1½ cups
1 sprig of thyme
1 tablespoon fresh or
   1 teaspoon dried oregano
⅓ cup fat-free sour cream
1 tablespoon cornstarch
   (tolerated), diluted in
   2 tablespoons water
2¼ lbs. clams, washed
   thoroughly

Finely chop the shallots and gently cook them in a saucepan with 4 tablespoons water until softened. Turn up the heat and add the tomatoes, herbs, sour cream, and the diluted cornstarch. Reduce for about 5 minutes.

Add the clams, and cook over medium heat until the clams open, about 7 minutes.

Serve with the vegetables of your choice.

Rabbit with a mustard sauce
and braised chicory

4 servings

Preparation time

  15 minutes

Cooking time

  55 minutes

1 teaspoon oil (tolerated)
1 rabbit, cut into pieces (you
  could also use a 3½-lb.
  chicken)
2 shallots, finely chopped
2¼ cups low-salt stock, with the
  fat skimmed off
3 tablespoons mustard (Dijon or
  whole-grain)
2 tablespoons fat-free sour
  cream
1 pinch of ground ginger
2 teaspoons chopped parsley
1 teaspoon finely chopped garlic
2 sprigs of rosemary
Salt and freshly ground black
  pepper

For the chicory
4 cups chicory or escarole
1 low-salt stock cube
Freshly ground black pepper
2 teaspoons chopped parsley
1 teaspoon finely chopped garlic

Using a paper towel, oil the bottom of a large frying pan. Over medium-high heat, place the rabbit pieces in the pan and sear them on all sides. Add the shallots, stirring until they turn golden brown. Pour in ½ cup water and the stock, add some salt and black pepper, cover and leave to simmer for 10 minutes.

Add the mustard, sour cream, ginger, parsley, garlic, and rosemary. Stir well with a wooden spoon. Cook for 15 minutes more.

While the rabbit is simmering, prepare the chicory. Cut the chicory into ¾-inch slices, wash and place on a clean kitchen towel to absorb the water. Then put the chicory slices in a sauté pan and cook over low heat until soft. Crumble in the stock cube and add ½ cup water. Season with pepper and finish off with the chopped parsley and garlic. Simmer until all the water has evaporated.

Serve the rabbit and mustard sauce with a spoonful of the braised chicory or escarole.

Asian-style mussels

2 servings

Preparation time

10 minutes

Cooking time

10 minutes

2¼ lbs. mussels
1 (6-oz.) can tomato paste
2 shallots, finely chopped
1 teaspoon ground cumin
1 pinch of ground ginger
½ bunch of parsley, chopped

Scrub the mussels and rinse well, discarding any that are broken or open.

Cover the mussels halfway with water in a large pan and stir in the tomato paste.

Add the shallots, cumin, ginger, and half the chopped parsley, and cook over high heat 3 to 7 minutes, until they open up (discard any that have not opened).

Sprinkle with the remaining parsley, and serve immediately.

Aniseed-flavored veal stew with fennel

4 servings

Preparation time

35 minutes

Cooking time

1 hour 15 minutes

4 fennel bulbs
1 large onion
4 carrots
1 leek, white part only
1¾ lbs. veal, trimmed of any fat
1 low-salt stock cube
2 whole cloves
2 star anise
2 bay leaves
Salt and freshly ground black
  pepper
2 tablespoons cornstarch
  (tolerated)
1 small or ½ large butternut
  squash
1 teaspoon curry powder

Remove the hard root end at the base of each fennel bulb.

Peel and finely chop the onion. Peel and thinly slice the carrots. Cut the fennel and leek into thin strips. Place the vegetables in a colander and wash them. Slice the veal into chunks, about 1 inch.

In a nonstick frying pan, gently cook the veal and onion. As soon as the veal starts to brown, cover it with water and crumble in the stock cube. Stir thoroughly. Add the vegetables, cloves, star anise, and bay leaves. Season with salt and pepper and bring to a boil. Stir, then simmer over low heat for 1 hour. At the last moment, stir in the cornstarch. Taste and, if necessary, adjust the seasoning.

In the meantime, remove the skin from the butternut squash and cut into ½-inch cubes. Cook the squash in a nonstick frying pan over medium heat with a little water in the bottom for 30 to 40 minutes. Add more water when necessary. When cooked, add the curry powder and season with salt and pepper. Use a fork to mash the squash a bit, leaving some chunks.

Serve the stew on warmed plates along with the butternut squash purée.

In the Consolidation phase, you can serve this stew with brown rice or couscous.

Carrot flan

4 servings

Preparation time
  15 minutes

Cooking time
  20 minutes

2 medium carrots
2 eggs
⅔ cup fat-free ricotta
¼ teaspoon nutmeg
¼ cup grated low fat Swiss or
  other hard cheese (tolerated)
Salt and freshly ground black
  pepper
1 teaspoon oil (tolerated)
2 teaspoons chopped parsley

Preheat oven to 475°F.

Peel, wash, and grate the carrots.

In a large bowl, whisk together the eggs, ricotta, nutmeg, and cheese. Add salt and pepper (you can also substitute different spices and use curry powder, cumin, etc.).

Using a paper towel, oil 4 ramekins (or 1 large ovenproof flan dish) and divide the grated carrots among them. Sprinkle each ramekin with 1 teaspoon of parsley. Divide the egg mixture among the ramekins.

Place the ramekins (or flan dish) on a baking sheet and bake for 20 minutes.

Let cool a little, then turn the flans out onto plates and sprinkle evenly with the remaining teaspoon of parsley. You may need a knife to turn them out.

This carrot flan is an excellent accompaniment for white meat.

Mushroom and tofu quiche

8 servings

Preparation time

20 minutes

Cooking time

45 minutes

1¼ lbs. mushrooms (if available, a mixture of button, shiitake, and oyster mushrooms)
1 teaspoon chopped parsley
Salt and freshly ground black pepper
1 (12.3-oz.) package silken tofu
4 eggs
½ cup grated low fat Swiss or other hard cheese (tolerated)
½ teaspoon nutmeg
8 cherry tomatoes

Preheat oven to 475°F.

Wipe the mushrooms clean with a paper towel. Slice them thinly and gently fry them in a nonstick frying pan with some parsley. Add salt and pepper to taste.

In the meantime, mix together in a bowl the tofu, eggs, cheese, and nutmeg. As soon as the mushrooms start to brown, add them to the tofu mixture. Stir thoroughly and adjust the seasoning, if necessary.

Pour the mixture into an ovenproof dish and arrange the cherry tomatoes on top, pushing them in slightly. Scatter a little parsley on top, if desired.

Bake for 40 minutes. Check the quiche and bake a little longer if not completely cooked.

This quiche goes well with a green salad.

Squash filled with veal Bolognese

4 servings

Preparation time

15 minutes

Cooking time

50 minutes

2 red kuri or acorn squash
1 onion
14 ozs. ground veal or lean
  ground beef
1 (6-oz.) can tomato paste
½ teaspoon mild chili powder
1 generous pinch of ground
  ginger
1 teaspoon chopped parsley
Salt and freshly ground black
  pepper

Preheat oven to 475°F.

Cut both squash lengthwise and, using a spoon, scoop out the seeds. Bake the squash halves on a rimmed baking sheet, cut side down, for 20 minutes.

In the meantime, peel and finely chop the onion and mix it with the ground veal or beef. Gently fry in a nonstick frying pan and, as soon as the meat is browned, add the tomato paste, spices, and parsley. Season with salt and pepper to taste.

Once the squash halves are cooked through, take them out of the oven and fill them with the veal Bolognese.

Bake the filled squash on the rimmed baking sheet for 30 minutes. Serve immediately.

Curried chicken club sandwich

2 servings

Preparation time

15 minutes

Cooking time

15 minutes

For the Dukan sandwich bread
3 generous tablespoons oat bran
1 teaspoon baking powder
2 tablespoons fat-free ricotta
1 egg
2 egg whites

1 large onion
½ teaspoon curry powder
1 large tomato
A few lettuce leaves
2 tablespoons fat-free cream
   cheese or 4 slices cheddar (in
   the Consolidation phase)
A little sugar-free ketchup
2 slices of cooked chicken

In a bowl, combine all the bread ingredients in the following order: the oat bran, baking powder, ricotta, egg, and egg whites. Pour this mixture into 2 small round baking dishes. Microwave for 5 minutes and leave to cool.

Peel and thinly slice the onion. In a frying pan, cook in a little water with the curry powder.

Wash and slice the tomato. Wash and dry the lettuce leaves.

As soon as the bread circles have cooled, remove them from the baking dishes, slice them in half, and toast them on the highest setting.

Put 2 of the bread halves on each plate. Spread 1 tablespoon of cream cheese (or 2 slices of cheese) on each "bottom" slice of bread. On each "bottom," add a little ketchup, then stack the curry-flavored onion slices, sliced tomato, and lettuce leaves. Add some sliced cooked chicken, and place the other bread halves on top and serve.

In the Attack phase, remember that you should not eat more than 1½ tablespoons of oat bran per day, and in the Cruise and Consolidation phases you should not eat more than 2 tablespoons of oat bran per day.

Chili con carne with tofu

2 servings

Preparation time

10 minutes

Cooking time

25 minutes

2 garlic cloves
2 onions
1 (12.3-oz.) package firm tofu
2 green chilies
14 oz. lean ground beef
2 (6-oz.) cans tomato paste
  mixed with 1 cup water
1 tablespoon chili powder
1 bay leaf
¼ teaspoon ground cumin
Salt and freshly ground black
  pepper

Chop the garlic, cut the onions into small pieces, crumble the tofu, and dice the green chilies. Sauté the vegetables and tofu with the beef in a nonstick frying pan for 5 minutes. Add remaining ingredients and mix thoroughly. Season with salt and pepper to taste.

When the ingredients come to a boil, cover, lower the heat slightly, and simmer for 15 minutes.

This dish could be served with some steamed zucchini or a green salad.

Eggplant and tofu lasagna

2 servings

Preparation time
25 minutes

Resting time
30 minutes

Cooking time
35 minutes

1 medium eggplant
Salt
1 zucchini
1 or 2 tomatoes
½ cup firm tofu (herb-flavored, if you can find it)
1 onion
1 garlic clove
½ low-salt chicken stock cube
1 teaspoon Italian herb seasoning
¼ cup grated low fat Swiss or other hard cheese, divided (tolerated)

Cut the eggplant into thin slices, sprinkle them with salt, and let drain for at least 30 minutes. Rinse the eggplant slices in cold water and pat dry.

Preheat oven to 475°F.

Thinly slice the zucchini and tomatoes. Cut the tofu into thin slices, and then finely chop the onion and garlic.

In a nonstick frying pan, cook the eggplant slices in 4 tablespoons water with the crumbled half stock cube for a few minutes until they turn slightly brown.

Do the same with the zucchini slices and tofu in separate pans. Set aside.

Gently cook the onion and garlic for 1 to 2 minutes in 2 tablespoons water. Add the tomato. Sprinkle in the Italian herb seasoning.

In an ovenproof dish, arrange the eggplant slices so that they completely cover the bottom. Place the zucchini on top of the eggplant. Make another layer with the tofu slices and scatter 2 tablespoons of the cheese on top. Add the tomato, onion, and garlic. Bake for 25 minutes.

Five minutes before the lasagna is ready to come out of the oven, sprinkle the remaining cheese over the top.

Stir-fried beef with sweet peppers

2 servings

Preparation time

15 minutes

Cooking time

20 minutes

2 red peppers
1 green pepper
14 ozs. flank steak
2 shallots, finely chopped
1 teaspoon low-sodium soy
  sauce
Salt and freshly ground black
  pepper
Some herbes de Provence (a
  mix of dried marjoram, thyme,
  savory, basil, rosemary, sage,
  and fennel seeds)

Halve the peppers, remove the ribs and seeds, and thinly slice them. Slice the beef into cubes.

In a large nonstick frying pan, gently fry the shallots and beef cubes for 5 to 10 minutes. Season with salt.

Add the peppers and cook for 10 minutes more, stirring constantly.

Two minutes before you are ready to serve, add the soy sauce.

Season with salt and pepper to taste, and sprinkle the herbs over the top.

Sea bass fillets with basil

3 servings

Preparation time

15 minutes

Cooking time

10 minutes

3 tomatoes
1 garlic clove
1 bunch of fresh basil
2 teaspoons olive oil (tolerated)
6 (3-oz.) sea bass fillets, or
   other firm white fish
1 tablespoon balsamic vinegar
Salt and freshly ground black
   pepper

Wash the tomatoes and chop them into small, even pieces. Peel the garlic. Wash and dry the basil and remove the leaves from the stems. Discard the stems.

Chop the basil leaves roughly in a blender, adding the garlic and 1 teaspoon of the olive oil. Set aside.

Pat the fish fillets dry with paper towels. Using a pastry brush, brush them all over with the rest of the olive oil. Heat a nonstick frying pan on high and fry the fillets for 2 minutes on each side. Season with salt. Remove the fillets from the pan and keep warm.

Pour the vinegar into the frying pan and use a spatula to scrape the pan and dissolve the cooking juices. Simmer for 1 minute. Add the tomatoes. Heat for 2 minutes in the cooking juices in the pan, stirring well so that the tomatoes get completely covered with the juices. Purée the sauce in a blender and season with salt and pepper to taste.

Transfer the tomato purée to a large serving dish. Arrange the fish fillets on top. Drizzle with the basil purée. Serve immediately.

Chicken, apple, and vegetable curry

2 servings

Preparation time

20 minutes

Cooking time

1 hour

1 eggplant
2 zucchini
2 onions
1 teaspoon olive oil (tolerated)
1 low-salt chicken stock cube
2 teaspoons curry powder
2 teaspoons chopped parsley
1 teaspoon finely chopped garlic
Salt and freshly ground black
    pepper
2 boneless, skinless chicken
    breasts
1 apple
1 pinch of ginger
⅓ cup fat-free sour cream

Wash and dice the eggplant and zucchini. Peel and finely chop 1 onion.

Sauté the vegetables for 10 minutes in a non-stick frying pan with the olive oil and 4 table-spoons water. If the vegetables start to stick, add a little more water.

Crumble in one half of the stock cube and add enough water to cover. Stir well and add 1 teaspoon curry powder along with the chopped parsley and garlic. Season with salt and pepper. Simmer on low heat for 20 min-utes, adding a little more water if necessary.

Slice the chicken breasts into strips. Peel and finely chop the remaining onion. Peel the apple and slice it thinly.

Cook the onion and apple in a nonstick fry-ing pan with 4 tablespoons water. As soon as they have softened, crumble in the other half of the stock cube and add 4 tablespoons water. Add the chicken strips and let them cook through, then stir in the remaining curry powder and ginger. Simmer for 10 minutes. Season with salt and pepper to taste.

Just before serving, mix the vegetables and chicken together and stir in the sour cream.

Normandy-style scallops

2 servings

Preparation time
  20 minutes

Cooking time
  20 minutes

4 teaspoons mustard
1 small bunch of fresh herbs,
  finely chopped
Salt and freshly ground black
  pepper
2 tomatoes
1 large apple
10½ ozs. bay or sea scallops
2 shallots, finely chopped
1 pinch of paprika
Juice of 1 lemon
2 tablespoons fat-free sour
  cream
1 teaspoon chopped parsley

Preheat oven to 350°F.

Mix together the mustard and fresh herbs with some salt and pepper.

Cut a thin lid off the top of the tomatoes and place them in an ovenproof dish. Divide the herb mixture between the tomatoes, put their lids back on, and bake for 20 minutes.

In the meantime, peel and slice the apple.

In a nonstick frying pan, gently fry the scallops with the sliced apple until lightly browned. Add the finely chopped shallots and season with salt, pepper, and paprika. Stir in the lemon juice and sour cream. Reduce the sauce, slightly, over very low heat.

Arrange the scallops on warmed plates, sprinkle with the chopped parsley, and serve with the baked tomatoes.

Coconut chicken with green beans and tofu

2 servings

Preparation time

10 minutes

Cooking time

15 minutes

2 boneless, skinless chicken breasts
⅔ cup coconut milk
1 teaspoon curry powder
½ cup firm tofu
Salt and freshly ground black pepper
2 handfuls of green beans (about 30 beans total)
A few long chives
A few sesame and poppy seeds (tolerated)

Slice the chicken breasts into cubes and cook in a nonstick frying pan until just browned. Add the coconut milk and curry powder, and simmer until cooked through. Set aside.

Dice the tofu and gently sauté it in a frying pan until lightly browned. Add some salt, pepper, and 2 tablespoons of the coconut sauce from the chicken pan, and cook 2 minutes more.

Meanwhile, remove both ends from the green beans and cook in salted boiling water until tender. When just cool enough to handle, tie the beans into 2 bundles using lengths of chives.

Arrange the chicken on plates with the curry coconut milk sauce, then add the tofu cubes.

Serve with the green bean bundles and, as a finishing touch, sprinkle a few sesame and poppy seeds over the tofu cubes.

Chicken and shrimp in a spicy coconut sauce

2 servings

Preparation time

20 minutes

Cooking time

20 minutes

1 boneless, skinless chicken
  breast
10½ ozs. shrimp, peeled and
  deveined, tails left on
2 garlic cloves
1 onion
1 teaspoon curry powder
½ teaspoon mild chili powder
Salt and freshly ground black
  pepper
⅔ cup coconut milk
6 white or green asparagus
  spears, cooked

Cut the chicken breast into pieces and fry over a gentle heat in a nonstick frying pan with a little water in the bottom of the pan. As soon as the water has evaporated, add the shrimp. Cook over low heat for 1 minute, stirring constantly with a wooden spoon.

Peel the garlic and onion. Finely chop them in a small food processor.

Put 4 tablespoons water in another frying pan and add the garlic/onion mixture. Heat gently for 1 minute and add the spices. Season with salt and pepper to taste. Pour in the coconut milk and simmer for 5 minutes, stirring occasionally.

Add the shrimp and chicken pieces, stirring to combine. Cook for 5 minutes over low heat.

Heat the asparagus either for 5 minutes in a frying pan or in a microwave for 1 minute.

Arrange the asparagus on 2 plates and spoon the chicken and shrimp mixture over the top. Serve immediately.

DESSERTS

Muesli ice cream

2 servings

Preparation time

15 minutes

Cooking time

15 minutes

Freezing and cooling time

4½ hours

½ vanilla bean
1 cup fat-free milk
4 tablespoons oat bran
2 tablespoons zero-calorie
    sweetener, suitable for
    cooking, such as Splenda
1 egg, beaten
1 tablespoon fat-free ricotta
1 tablespoon fat-free plain Greek-
    style yogurt
⅛ teaspoon orange-flower water
    or a ½ teaspoon of grated
    orange zest

Split the half vanilla bean lengthwise, scrape out the seeds, and place them in a saucepan with the milk. Bring the milk to a boil. Remove the pan from heat and add the oat bran and 1 tablespoon of the sweetener. Stir carefully to combine, then place the pan back over low heat and allow the bran mixture to thicken. Stir in the beaten egg, combine thoroughly, then remove the pan from heat. Remove the vanilla bean.

In a large bowl, mix together the ricotta, yogurt, remaining sweetener, and orange flavoring. Stir in the bran mixture.

Pour the mixture into 2 glasses and let cool to room temperature, about 30 minutes.

When cool, put the glasses in the freezer for at least 4 hours. Stir the ice cream every hour to prevent crystals from forming.

In the Attack phase, remember you should not eat more than 1½ tablespoons of oat bran per day, and in the Cruise and Consolidation phases you should not eat more than 2 tablespoons of oat bran per day.

Fluffy pistachio mousse

8 to 10 servings

Preparation time

15 minutes

Cooking time

5 minutes

Refrigeration time

4 hours

1½ (7-gram) envelopes
(10½ grams total) unflavored
gelatin
2 to 3 tablespoons zero-calorie
sweetener, suitable for cooking
and baking, such as Splenda
2 teaspoons pistachio
flavor extract (optional) or
peppermint extract (for mint
mousse)
5 drops of natural green food
coloring (optional)
4 egg whites
1 pinch of salt
1⅓ cups fat-free ricotta

Dissolve the gelatin in 2 tablespoons cold water.

Put the sweetener in a saucepan and add 4 tablespoons water. Bring to a boil and let boil for 2 minutes. Add the pistachio or peppermint extract, gelatin, and food coloring, if using. Stir well and remove from heat.

In a bowl, whisk the egg whites and a pinch of salt until stiff. Slowly drizzle in the flavored syrup, whisking constantly. Gently fold the egg whites into the ricotta, taking care not to break up the eggs.

Divide the mixture among 8 to 10 small glasses and refrigerate for 4 hours before serving.

Consuming raw or undercooked eggs carries the risk of serious food poisoning with salmonella bacteria. Raw or undercooked eggs should not be eaten by the very young, the very old, pregnant women, or anyone with a compromised immune system.

Iced chocolate soufflés

8 servings

Preparation time

15 minutes

Cooking time

5 minutes

Freezing time

8 hours

1½ (7-gram) envelopes
(10½ grams total) unflavored
gelatin
½ cup low-fat cocoa powder
(tolerated)
1 teaspoon coffee flavor extract
(optional) or very strong coffee
2 eggs, separated
1 pinch of salt
½ cup plus 2 tablespoons fat-
free ricotta
4 tablespoons zero-calorie
sweetener, suitable for cooking
and baking, such as Splenda

Dissolve the gelatin in 2 tablespoons cold water.

In a saucepan, gently warm the cocoa powder with 3 tablespoons water and the coffee extract. Remove from heat and add the 2 egg yolks and the gelatin.

In a bowl, whisk the egg whites and a pinch of salt until stiff.

Using a whisk, blend the ricotta and sweetener, and then add the cocoa mixture. Stir together thoroughly and gently fold in the whisked egg whites. Pour this mixture into 8 glasses, molds, or ramekins. Freeze for 8 hours.

Take the soufflés out of the freezer 10 minutes before you are ready to serve.

Tofu chocolate cream

6 to 8 servings

Preparation time

5 minutes

Refrigeration time

1 hour

1 cup silken tofu
¼ cup fat-free ricotta
10 ozs. fat-free vanilla yogurt
2 teaspoons low-fat cocoa
  powder (tolerated)
2 tablespoons zero-calorie
  sweetener, such as Splenda
  (or more according to taste)

Using a whisk or hand mixer on medium speed blend together the tofu, ricotta, yogurt, cocoa powder, and sweetener until the mixture is smooth and creamy.

Pour the mixture into glasses and refrigerate for 1 hour before serving.

St. Tropez tart

6 servings

Preparation time

25 minutes

Cooking and cooling time

2 hours

For the brioche
3 tablespoons oat bran
1 tablespoon cornstarch
  (tolerated)
1 tablespoon skim milk powder
2 eggs
1 cup fat-free yogurt
1 tablespoon fat-free Greek-style
  yogurt
1 tablespoon fat-free ricotta
1 teaspoon baking powder
2 tablespoons zero-calorie
  sweetener, suitable for cooking
  and baking, such as Splenda
1½ teaspoons orange-flower
  water

For the filling
2 (7-gram) envelopes unflavored
  gelatin, divided
1 vanilla bean
2¼ cups fat-free milk, divided
3 eggs, separated
2 tablespoons zero-calorie
  sweetener, such as Splenda
2 tablespoons cornstarch
  (tolerated)
1 tablespoon rum flavoring
  (optional)
1 pinch of salt

Preheat oven to 350°F.

Combine all the brioche ingredients and pour the batter into a silicone mold. Bake for 20 minutes. Cool, then slice the cake into two layers.

Dissolve 1 envelope of the gelatin in ¼ cup of the milk.

Split the vanilla bean lengthwise, scrape out the seeds, and place the bean and seeds in a saucepan with the remaining milk. Bring to a boil.

In the meantime, mix together the egg yolks, sweetener, cornstarch, and rum flavoring in a bowl. Reserve the egg whites for later.

Remove the milk from the heat, take out the vanilla pod, and stir in the gelatin. Pour the milk over the egg mixture, stirring carefully all the time. Pour it all back into a saucepan and let the mixture thicken, stirring with a wooden spoon. Before the mixture comes to a boil and as it starts to thicken, remove the pan from the heat. Set aside to cool.

Dissolve the remaining envelope of gelatin in 1 tablespoon water.

Whisk the egg whites with a pinch of salt until very firm. Add the gelatin.

Fold the egg whites into the egg mixture and set in a cool place for 1 hour, then spread it over 1 cake half. Place the other cake half on top.

Gingerbread

6 to 8 servings

Preparation time

10 minutes

Cooking time

45 minutes

¾ cup oat bran
2 tablespoons powdered skim milk
2 teaspoons baking powder
6 tablespoons fat-free ricotta
3 eggs
3 egg whites
2 tablespoons gingerbread spice mix (cinnamon, aniseed, nutmeg, ginger, cloves)
1 tablespoon zero-calorie sweetener, suitable for cooking and baking, such as Splenda, dissolved in 1 tablespoon water
1 teaspoon vegetable oil (tolerated)

Preheat oven to 350°F.

Oil an ovenproof dish, wiping out the excess with a paper towel.

In a bowl, combine the oat bran, powdered milk, and baking powder. Add the ricotta, stir thoroughly and then add the eggs and 3 egg whites. Keep stirring until the mixture is smooth, then add the spices and sweetener. Pour the batter into the ovenproof dish.

Bake for 45 minutes, or until a toothpick inserted in the center comes out clean.

In the Attack phase, remember that you should not eat more than 1½ tablespoons of oat bran per day, and during the Cruise phase you should not eat more than 2 tablespoons of oat bran per day.

Ricotta clementine creams

6 servings

Preparation time

20 minutes

Cooking time

30 minutes

Refrigeration time

5 hours

2 (7-gram) envelopes unflavored gelatin

3½ cups fat-free milk, divided

2 vanilla beans

Zest of 2 clementines, satsumas, or tangerines (unwaxed if possible)

1 teaspoon cinnamon

4 egg yolks

4 tablespoons zero-calorie sweetener, suitable for cooking and baking, such as Splenda (or more according to taste)

1 cup fat-free ricotta

½ cup fat-free sour cream (optional)

1 tablespoon orange extract (optional)

Dissolve the gelatin in ½ cup of the milk.

Split the vanilla beans lengthwise, scrape out the seeds, and place them in a saucepan with the remaining 3 cups milk, zest from the clementines, and cinnamon. Bring to a boil, remove from heat, and let infuse, covered, for 20 minutes.

In a large bowl, whisk together the egg yolks, the sweetener, ricotta, sour cream, and orange extract.

Using a small conical strainer, pour the milk over the egg yolk mixture, discard the beans, and stir vigorously. Warm the mixture in a pan over low heat, stirring constantly with a wooden spoon, until the cream is thick enough to coat the back of the spoon.

Remove from heat and stir in the gelatin. Pour the mixture into 6 dishes or ramekins. Let cool to room temperature, then refrigerate for 5 hours.

Serve plain in the Cruise phase, or with clementine segments in the Consolidation phase.

As a variation, use pistachio flavoring with the grated zest from 1 lemon.

Grand Marnier Swiss roll

6 servings

Preparation time

15 minutes

Cooking time

25 minutes

Refrigeration time

2 hours

1 (7-gram) envelope unflavored gelatin
1 cup plus 2 tablespoons fat-free milk, divided
2 egg yolks
1 tablespoon zero-calorie sweetener, suitable for cooking and baking, such as Splenda
1 tablespoon cornstarch (tolerated)
1 teaspoon orange-flower water or some grated orange zest

For the sponge cake
3 eggs, separated
3 tablespoons oat bran
1 tablespoon skim milk powder
2 tablespoons fat-free plain Greek-style yogurt
2 tablespoons fat-free ricotta
1 tablespoon cornstarch (tolerated)
1 teaspoon baking powder
1 teaspoon vanilla extract
2 tablespoons zero-calorie sweetener, suitable for cooking and baking

Dissolve the gelatin in 2 tablespoons milk.

Heat 1 cup milk to a boil. Mix together the egg yolks, sweetener, cornstarch, and orange-flower water in a bowl. Remove the milk from the heat and add the gelatin, stirring thoroughly. Carefully pour the milk over the egg mixture, stirring constantly with a wooden spoon. Pour the mixture back into a saucepan and let thicken over low heat. Remove from heat and cool to room temperature, then refrigerate for 2 hours.

While the cream is chilling, start the sponge cake. Preheat oven to 325°F. Beat the egg whites until stiff. Set aside. Put the egg yolks in a bowl and stir in the oat bran, milk powder, yogurt, ricotta, cornstarch, baking powder, vanilla, and sweetener, and whisk together vigorously. Fold in the beaten egg whites. Spread the batter on a silicone Swiss roll pan (turning out the cake is easier with silicone). Bake until the cake turns golden brown. Turn the cake out onto a damp kitchen towel and immediately roll it up. Let cool, then unroll the cake. Spread the cream over the cake, and very gently roll it up again.

In the Consolidation phase, you could spread a little apricot jam (see page 228) on the sponge cake before rolling up with the cream.

In the Attack phase, remember that you should not eat more than 1½ tablespoons of oat bran per day, and during the Cruise phase you should not eat more than 2 tablespoons of oat bran per day.

Rhubarb compote

6 servings

Preparation time

10 minutes

Resting time

15 minutes

Cooking time

30 minutes

2¼ lbs. rhubarb
6 tablespoons zero-calorie
   sweetener, suitable for cooking
   and baking, such as Splenda
   (or more according to taste)
10 drops of vanilla extract or
   another flavor (depending
   on the flavoring, try adding
   10 drops, taste and add more
   if required)

Quickly wash the rhubarb and without peeling it slice it into ½- to ¾-inch thick chunks.

Put the rhubarb chunks in a colander and sprinkle with the sweetener. Drain for 10 to 15 minutes, reserving the rhubarb liquid.

Cook over low heat in its own liquid, stirring frequently. Simmer for about 30 minutes, until you have the consistency you want. Once cooked, add the extract. Cool a little, then purée the compote in a food processor.

Lemon and lime mousse

6 servings

Preparation time
25 minutes

Cooking time
35 minutes

Refrigeration time
2 hours 30 minutes

For the candied fruit
4 tablespoons zero-calorie
  sweetener, suitable for cooking
  and baking, such as Splenda
1 lemon
1 lime

For the mousse
2 lemons
1 (7-gram) envelope unflavored
  gelatin
4 eggs, 2 separated
3 tablespoons zero-calorie
  sweetener, suitable for cooking
  and baking, such as Splenda
½ cup fat-free milk
1 pinch of salt
1 oat bran galette, (see
  page 48), crumbled

For the candied fruit, combine the sweetener with 1 cup water, warm over low heat, and set aside.

Cut the lemon and lime into very thin slices and remove any seeds. Cut the slices into quarters. Boil them in the syrup over low heat for 18 minutes. Cool, then strain. Put the candied lemon and lime on a plate. Reserve 2 tablespoons of syrup for the mousse.

To make the mousse, start by grating the lemon zest, then set it aside in a small dish. Juice the lemons into a bowl, reserve.

Dissolve the gelatin in 2 tablespoons water.

Whisk 2 eggs and 2 egg yolks with the sweetener until the mixture turns frothy. Set the 2 egg whites aside. Add the zest and lemon juice, put the mixture into a saucepan and let it thicken a little over low heat, stirring constantly. Pour in the milk gradually. Remove the pan from the heat and stir in the gelatin thoroughly.

Whisk the 2 egg whites with the pinch of salt until firm. When almost finished, gently fold in the reserved 2 tablespoons of syrup, then stir this into the lemon custard.

Refrigerate the mousse for at least 2½ hours before serving. Divide the crumbled galette among 6 serving cups. Top with mousse, and garnish each portion with candied lemon and lime before serving.

Vanilla-hazelnut crème brûlée with strawberries

6 servings

Preparation time

15 minutes

Cooking time

40 minutes

Refrigeration time

1 hour

2¼ cups fat-free milk
1 vanilla bean
4 egg yolks
6 tablespoons zero-calorie
  sweetener, suitable for cooking
  and baking, such as Splenda
½ teaspoon hazelnut extract
  (optional)
12 fresh strawberries
⅔ cup fat-free sour cream

Pour the milk into a saucepan, split the vanilla bean in half lengthwise, scrape out the seeds, and add them to the milk. Bring to a boil. Remove from heat, cover, and infuse for 5 to 10 minutes. Remove and discard the vanilla bean.

Preheat oven to 350°F.

Beat the egg yolks with the sweetener and hazelnut extract, if using.

Slice the strawberries and arrange them in 6 large ramekins or shallow dishes.

Stir the hot milk thoroughly into the egg yolk mixture, and then add the sour cream. Pour this mixture over the strawberries and bake for 30 minutes.

Cool the brûlées to room temperature, then refrigerate for 1 hour before serving.

Lemony mousse

6 servings

Preparation time
15 minutes

Cooking time
20 minutes

Refrigeration time
30 minutes

3 lemons
3 eggs, separated
3 tablespoons zero-calorie
  sweetener, suitable for cooking
  and baking, such as Splenda
  (or more according to taste)
3 tablespoons cornstarch
  (tolerated)
2¼ cups fat-free milk

Zest 1 lemon. Juice all 3 lemons.

Put the lemon zest and juice in a sauce-pan and add the egg yolks and sweetener. Combine thoroughly, then gradually stir in the cornstarch.

Heat the mixture, stirring constantly with a wooden spoon. Let it thicken, and then grad-ually add the milk. Stir well and let it thicken some more. Remove the pan from the heat and set it aside to cool.

Whisk the egg whites until very firm and gen-tly fold them into the cooled lemon custard. Pour the mousse into 6 glasses or ramekins and refrigerate for 30 minutes before serving.

Pineapple with iced crème anglaise

2 servings

Preparation time

15 minutes

Cooking time

20 minutes

Freezing time

3 hours

1 vanilla bean
1 cup fat-free milk
3 egg yolks
3 tablespoons zero-calorie
  sweetener, suitable for cooking
  and baking, such as Splenda
20 drops of rum extract
  (optional)
2 large slices of pineapple, cut
  in half

Split the vanilla bean lengthwise, scrape out the seeds, and place them in a saucepan with the milk. Bring to a boil and let infuse for 10 minutes. Remove from heat and discard vanilla bean.

In a large bowl, whisk together the egg yolks with the sweetener and rum extract, if using. Pour the hot milk over the egg yolk mixture, stirring vigorously. Warm the mixture over low heat, stirring constantly with a wooden spoon until the crème covers the back of the spoon. Pour the crème into 2 glasses.

Cool to room temperature, and then freeze for 3 hours.

Garnish with pineapple slices, and serve.

Apricot clafoutis

6 servings

Preparation time

   10 minutes

Cooking time

   45 minutes

4 eggs
2 tablespoons whole wheat flour
2 cups fat-free milk
3 tablespoons zero-calorie
   sweetener, suitable for cooking
   and baking, such as Splenda
1 teaspoon baking powder
2 tablespoons pistachio extract
   (optional)
14 ripe apricots

Preheat oven to 350°F.

Beat the eggs, then stir in the flour, milk, sweetener, baking powder, and extract, if using.

Halve the apricots, remove the pits, and arrange the halves in rows in 1 nonstick dish or 6 small dishes. Pour the egg mixture over the top.

Bake for 45 minutes. Check to see if the clafoutis is ready and, if necessary, bake a little longer.

Let the clafoutis cool to room temperature before serving.

Spicy compote

4 servings

Preparation time

25 minutes

Cooking time

30 minutes

1 orange
4 medium apples
1 cinnamon stick
1 clove
2 cardamom pods
3 tablespoons oat bran

Peel the orange and cut it into quarters.

Peel and core the apples and cut them into small cubes.

Lightly toast the cinnamon, clove, and seeds from the cardamom pods in a clean nonstick frying pan. Then add the orange quarters and apple cubes.

Cook, covered, over medium heat for about 30 minutes, until the apples start to break down.

Sprinkle with the oat bran, and serve.

Vanilla panna cotta with raspberries and balsamic syrup

4 servings

Preparation time

15 minutes

Cooking time

20 minutes

Refrigeration time

8 hours

2 (7-gram) envelopes unflavored gelatin
2 vanilla beans
2¼ cups fat-free milk, divided
4 egg yolks
4 tablespoons zero-calorie sweetener, suitable for cooking and baking, such as Splenda
⅔ cup fat-free sour cream
A drizzle of balsamic vinegar glaze made by reducing balsamic vinegar until thickened (the smell is very strong, so ventilate the kitchen well)
20 fresh raspberries (or more if you really enjoy them)

Dissolve the gelatin in ¼ cup milk.

Split the vanilla beans lengthwise, scrape out the seeds, and place them in a saucepan with the remaining 2 cups milk. Bring the mixture to a boil.

In a bowl, whisk together the egg yolks with 2 tablespoons of the sweetener.

Remove and discard the vanilla beans, and pour the milk over the egg yolks, stirring constantly. Put the mixture back in the pan, and warm over low heat, stirring constantly with a wooden spoon, until the custard is thick enough to coat the spoon.

Remove the pan from heat and stir in the gelatin mixture. Cool to room temperature.

In a bowl, whisk together the sour cream and remaining 2 tablespoons of sweetener, then add the egg mixture. Pour the panna cotta into 4 small molds or ramekins, and cool to room temperature. Refrigerate for 8 hours.

When ready to serve, turn the panna cottas carefully out onto plates, drizzle with the balsamic vinegar glaze, and garnish with the raspberries.

Strawberry and vanilla soy pudding

2 servings

Preparation time

10 minutes

Refrigeration time

10 minutes

10 medium, fresh strawberries
½ lemon, juiced
Zero-calorie sweetener, suitable
for cooking and baking, such
as Splenda (more or less,
according to taste)
1 cup vanilla-flavored soy yogurt
or plain soy yogurt with vanilla
and sweetener

Hull the strawberries, and purée them with the lemon juice and the sweetener. Taste, add more sweetener if necessary, and refrigerate for 10 minutes.

Pour some of the strawberry purée into 2 glasses. Add a layer of yogurt, another layer of purée, and then finish with the remaining yogurt.

Apricot jam

Makes 1 jar

Preparation time

15 minutes

Cooking time

15 minutes

10½ ozs. ripe apricots
4 tablespoons zero-calorie
sweetener, suitable for cooking
and baking, such as Splenda
(more or less, according to
taste)
1 pinch of cinnamon
¾ teaspoon unflavored gelatin

Wash the apricots, cut into quarters, and re-move the pits. Put them in a saucepan with the sweetener and cinnamon. Bring to a boil, decrease the heat to low, and simmer for 5 minutes.

Slowly add the gelatin, stirring constantly, and cook for 1 minute. Gently mash the mix-ture with a fork.

Immediately pour the jam into a sterilized jar, seal using some plastic wrap and a rubber band, then affix a lid. Store in the refrigerator.

Floating islands with a hint of mocha

4 servings

Preparation time

15 minutes

Cooking time

20 minutes

Refrigeration time

1 hour

4 eggs, separated
1 teaspoon coffee extract
   (optional) or very strong coffee
4 tablespoons zero-calorie
   sweetener, suitable for cooking
   and baking, such as Splenda,
   divided
1 vanilla bean or 1 teaspoon
   vanilla extract
½ cup low-fat evaporated milk
½ cup fat-free milk
1 to 2 teaspoons cornstarch
   (tolerated)

In a bowl, whisk the egg whites, coffee extract, if using, and 2 tablespoons of the sweetener until firm.

Using a tablespoon, shape the egg whites into small meringues, and microwave them on high for 1 minute. Place the cooked meringues on paper towels to cool to room temperature.

Split the vanilla bean lengthwise, if using, scrape out the seeds, and place them in a saucepan with the evaporated and fat-free milks. Bring the milk to a boil. Remove from the heat and discard the vanilla bean. Keep hot.

In a large bowl, mix together the egg yolks, the remaining 2 tablespoons of sweetener, and cornstarch. Gradually pour in the hot milk, and then return the mixture to the pan and warm over low heat. Stir with a wooden spoon until the custard is thick enough to coat the back of the spoon. Remove the pan from the heat and cool to room temperature. Refrigerate for 1 hour.

Divide the custard among 4 dessert dishes, reserving a few tablespoons for drizzling, then arrange the meringues on top. Drizzle the reserved custard over top of the meringues. Serve immediately.

Cinnamon apple surprise

4 servings

Preparation time

15 minutes

Cooking time

25 minutes

4 large Golden Delicious apples
1 egg
⅔ cup fat-free cottage cheese,
  drained
2 tablespoons zero-calorie
  sweetener, suitable for cooking
  and baking, such as Splenda
1 teaspoon cinnamon
1 teaspoon vanilla extract

Preheat oven to 350°F.

Core and cut the top off each apple. Scoop out some of the flesh without poking through the sides of the apples.

In a bowl, beat together the egg, cottage cheese, sweetener, cinnamon, and vanilla extract.

Fill the apples with the cottage-cheese mixture, put the tops back on the apples, and wrap each one in parchment paper.

Place on a baking sheet and bake for 25 minutes.

Serve warm.

Index

Bibliography

L'Complete Recipe Book des recettes Dukan
   Illustrées pour bien réussir la méthode,
   Flammarion, 2011
La pâtisserie Dukan, J'ai Lu, 2011
Les 100 aliments Dukan à volonté, J'ai Lu,
   2010

Le Guide nutritionnel Dukan des aliments
   santé & minceur, Le Cherche Midi, 2010

WEBSITE
www.dukandiet.com
www.shopdukandiet.com

Acknowledgments

My thanks go to all those people who throughout my life have helped me build this method. And most of all, I would like to thank my anonymous readers and patients who, of their own volition, have quite spontaneously gone about making the method known.

And among them, there is one who stands out: Carole Kitzinger. As talented as she is able, and yet so modest. Without her, this book would never have happened. Simone Gloger, thank you for your invaluable contribution to this book. I am grateful to you and your dedicated belief in my diet to end the obesity epidemic. Your support for this and future books continues to empower people in the United States and Canada. And since I am thanking people, I want to mention Vahinée, who knows my method perhaps better than I do. Also, a very big thank-you to Laura, who for several years has helped me day-to-day and who has worked alongside me to update this book.

Nathalie, Christine, Laetitia, Camelia, and Isabelle, names to you, but for me they are stars.

Dukan Diet Products

Oat bran: In addition to the standard form, our oat bran now comes in other forms, including coconut flavored and chocolate chip **oat bran cookies,** coconut almond and chocolate flavored **oat bran bars,** chocolate and vanilla **oat bran muffin mixes,** and more.

Low-fat cocoa is a great antioxidant and contains flavonoids that studies show support cardiovascular health. Low-fat cocoa allows you to produce a range of wonderful, light cakes and cookies without depriving yourself of the taste of chocolate while dieting.

Goji berries: There is quite a craze for these berries that originate from China, because they are naturally rich in vitamins, trace elements, and antioxidants. Many benefits are attributed to them, including strengthening the immune system, lowering blood pressure and blood glucose levels, and stimulating digestion. When dieting, they can aid with energy production and help to alleviate constipation.

Shirataki noodles: Shirataki noodles are cooked exactly like spaghetti. High in fiber, they absorb up to one hundred times their weight in water. These noodles have no particular taste and should be served in a well-seasoned, flavorful sauce, since they soak up the flavor of whatever they are combined with.

From the Attack phase onward, they can be eaten with Bolognese if you cut down on the amount of tomato sauce but keep to the quantity of ground beef. In the Cruise phase, you can then add to them all sorts of vegetables such as diced eggplant, zucchini, strips of sweet pepper, etc., and in the Consolidation phase you can add a little parmesan.

Dukan Diet Marinara Sauce: Dukan Diet Marinara Sauce is made with only premium, fresh, and natural ingredients. Prepared in small batches to slowly layer flavors for a true homemade taste, Dukan Diet Marinara Sauce can be used in many different recipes. From the Cruise phase on you can enjoy this marinara sauce on meats, fish, and vegetables, on oat bran pizza bases, and as a dip.

All these products are available at www.shopdukandiet.com.

Can't get enough of Dukan?

Discover the Complete Dukan Diet Library!

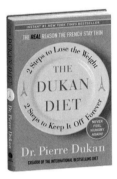

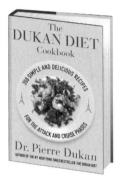

The Dukan Diet has helped millions of readers around the world to lose weight and keep it off.

The Dukan Diet Cookbook has 350 delicious recipes to help make losing weight a pleasure!

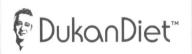
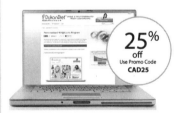
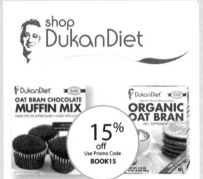

Portraits
of Sarajevo

Also by Zlatko Dizdarević:

SARAJEVO:
A War Journal